Autologous
Stem Cell Transplants

A Handbook for Patients

Did You Find This Book Helpful?

We strive to make our patient handbooks as comprehensive and easy-to-understand as possible. Your feedback helps keep us on track!

Please take a moment to let us know what you think about this book – what you like, what you don't like and how you believe we can improve it. It's input from people, like you, that will help make future editions of this book even more valuable for patients.

You can submit your comments online at www.bmtinfonet.org/bookcomments or phone us at 888-597-7674. We'd love to hear from you and help you in any other way that we can.

Other books written by Susan K. Stewart:

Bone Marrow & Blood Stem Cell Transplants:
A Guide for Patients and Their Loved Ones

ISBN 0-9647352-3-7
(for patients undergoing an allogeneic transplant)

Trasplantes de Médula Ósea y de
Células Progenitoras en Sangre Periférica:
Una Guía Para Pacientes

ISBN 0-9647352-4-5

Autologous Stem Cell Transplants

A Handbook for Patients

By Susan K. Stewart

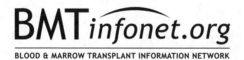

BLOOD & MARROW TRANSPLANT INFORMATION NETWORK

2310 Skokie Valley Road, Suite 104, Highland Park, IL 60035

phone: 847-433-3313   toll-free: 888-597-7674   fax: 847-433-4599

email: help@bmtinfonet.org

www.bmtinfonet.org

Publication of this book was made possible, in part, by a generous gift from

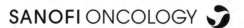

Acknowledgements

Writing this book was not a solo effort. The generosity of many wonderful people — doctors, nurses, social workers, transplant survivors, caregivers, my family and friends — is reflected in this book. They patiently shared with me their time, expertise and personal experiences. Without their help, this book would not have been possible.

Special thanks to:

Patrick J. Stiff MD, who contributed countless hours, providing me with background material, reviewing drafts of the book, responding to my many questions, and clarifying many technical details.

Martin S. Tallman MD, a warm, caring doctor and a personal friend who supported me first through my transplant, and afterwards as a medical advisor on this book.

Jan Sugar, who helped write and edit several sections of this book.

Norm Bendell, whose illustrations appear throughout the book. Thanks, Norm, for helping us lighten up a very difficult text.

The many medical professionals, too numerous to mention, who reviewed individual chapters or the final draft of the book.

The wonderful staff at BMT InfoNet—**Lynne Spina**, who helped with the writing, editing and production of this book; **Marla O'Keefe** and **Cindy Kessler** who reviewed and edited countless drafts; and **Kathy German**, who makes sure the book gets into the hands of every patient that needs it.

Kim Kultgen, our graphic designer, who spent many long hours coordinating the design and production of this book.

The transplant survivors quoted throughout the book, who gave it life. They have journeyed down the transplant path and have generously shared their experience and insights.

The caregivers who supported a loved one through a transplant, and are survivors in their own right. Thanks for generously sharing your stories and advice.

Thank you all!

This book is dedicated
to
Ruth Krueger
My mother, mentor and constant source of support

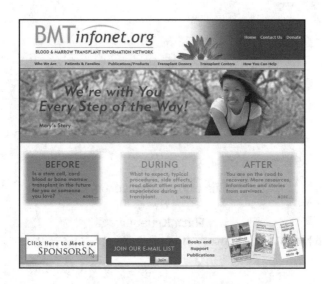

Visit www.bmtinfonet.org

For answers, advice and a caring companion throughout your transplant journey, visit bmtinfonet.org. Our web site is your gateway to detailed information about what to expect before, during and after your transplant. Popular features include:

- Detailed information about each step of the transplant process, potential complications and practical solutions

- Emotional support for patients, survivors and caregivers

- Facts about more than 200 transplant centers including staff, number of transplants performed, accreditation and diseases treated

- Extensive information for survivors about how to live well after transplant

You can also phone us toll free at 888-597-7674 for help.

We're with you every step of the way!

BMT InfoNet
Caring Connections
Program

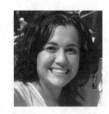

If you or a loved one is going to have a bone marrow, peripheral blood stem cell or cord blood transplant, chances are you are feeling scared and overwhelmed.

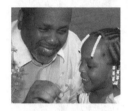

BMT InfoNet's **Caring Connections Program** can help.

More than 800 transplant survivors and their family members have volunteered to provide support to others facing a transplant.

Talk with people who:

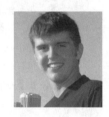

- have been through a transplant

- understand how you feel

- can provide non-medical information and emotional support

- can offer tips for coping with household and job responsibilities, the needs of other family members, and more.

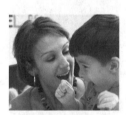

In most cases, our Caring Connections program can connect you with a survivor who had the same diagnosis, same type of transplant and is approximately the same age.

If you are a family member of a patient, you can use the Caring Connections program too!

Request a Caring Connection by phoning 888-597-7674 or online at www.bmtinfonet.org/services/support.

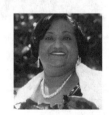

Someone in our community of volunteers is looking forward to talking with you!

Table of Contents

Appendices

Dear Friend,

In 1988, after being diagnosed with leukemia, my doctor recommended an autologous bone marrow transplant. I'd never before heard of a bone marrow transplant, and hadn't a clue as to what bone marrow or stem cells were and why they are important.

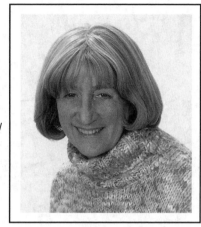

I was confused and overwhelmed. All the medical terms used to describe the treatment were new to me; often, I was so lost I couldn't even figure out the right questions to ask! After recovering from my transplant, I met other survivors and learned my experience was not unique.

This book is written by and for patients with the help of many doctors, nurses, social workers, survivors and their families. It's designed to translate, into plain English, the medical information you'll receive before, during and after your transplant.

There's no getting around it. Autologous transplantation is a big, confusing subject. There's a lot of information to absorb in this book. Take it at your own pace.

If you only want the basics, start with Chapters One and Two. Then use the table of contents and index to find answers to the questions that concern you the most. When you are ready for more details, read the other chapters that thoroughly discuss each step of the transplant process, how complications are managed, and how other patients have coped with the experience.

Throughout the book you will find quotations from transplant survivors — real people who faced the same challenges that now lie before you. They will tell you firsthand what it feels like to undergo and survive a transplant.

I know how difficult it is to make the decision to have an autologous transplant, undergo the treatment, and get back to a normal life. I hope this book helps make your experience a little easier.

Sue Stewart

Susan Stewart
Executive Director, BMT InfoNet

Chapter One
HISTORY OF TRANSPLANTATION

When I was first diagnosed with leukemia, I got very little encouragement from my local oncologist. Back then, bone marrow transplants weren't so common. He really tried to discourage me. He said 'A transplant is not for you. You might as well give up.' It felt pretty good to come home after my transplant, a survivor.

Jean Durko, 15-year transplant survivor

History and Use of Bone Marrow and Stem Cell Transplantation

Bone marrow, peripheral blood stem cell and umbilical cord blood transplantation are relatively new medical procedures used to treat diseases once thought incurable. Patients with diseases such as multiple myeloma, lymphoma, Hodgkin disease, autoimmue and genetic diseases and some solid tumors may be a candidate for an autologous transplant.

The technical name for bone marrow, peripheral blood stem cell and cord blood transplantation is hematopoietic cell transplantation.

Types of Transplants

There are three types of transplantation: allogeneic (al-o-je-náy-ik), syngeneic (sin-je-náy-ik) and autologous (aw-tól-o-gus).

Allogeneic transplantation is typically used to treat people who have a bone marrow disorder such as leukemia or aplastic anemia. In this procedure, the diseased bone marrow is destroyed by high-dose chemotherapy and/or radiation and replaced with blood stem cells provided by a donor.

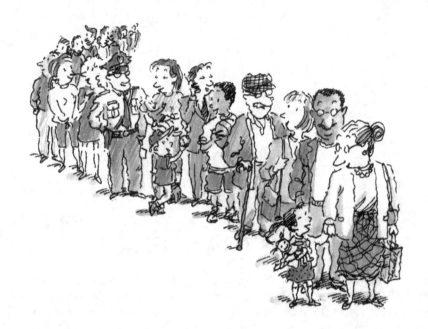

Syngeneic transplantation is similar to allogeneic transplantation. The difference is that with a syngeneic transplant, the donor is an identical twin, rather than another relative or an unrelated donor.

Autologous transplantation — the type of transplant being discussed in this book — is much more common today than allogeneic transplantation and involves fewer potential complications. In this procedure, the person's own stem cells are collected and stored. The patient then undergoes high-dose chemotherapy and/or radiation to destroy the disease, after which the stem cells are re-infused into the patient.

A Historical Perspective

The first serious attempts to transplant bone marrow into humans occurred in the late 1950s. Although several of the patients achieved a remission after transplant (there was no evidence of disease), most of them relapsed shortly thereafter.

The first successful bone marrow transplant took place in 1968. An infant with an immune deficiency disease was transplanted with bone marrow donated by a sibling. Similar successes soon were reported for patients with aplastic anemia and acute leukemia. By 1986, more than 200 transplant centers worldwide were performing 5,000 transplants annually.

Unfortunately, many patients who could have benefited from a bone marrow transplant could not undergo the procedure because they did not have a sibling with a matching marrow type. In 1973, a team of doctors in New York overcame this obstacle when they transplanted a five-year-old child who had severe combined immunodeficiency syndrome (SCIDS). The marrow was provided by an unrelated Danish donor. After seven transplants, the marrow engrafted and began producing normal blood cells. In 1986, the National Marrow Donor Registry® (now called the Be the Match Registry®) was established to facilitate more transplants with unrelated donors.

It was not until the late 1980s that autologous transplants became widely used. In 1978, researchers reported several successful autologous transplants in patients with lymphoma. By 1990, more autologous transplants were being performed than allogeneic transplants. An estimated 30,000 autologous transplants are now performed each year.

Diseases Treated

More than two dozen different diseases are now treated with autologous transplantation. Those treated most often are multiple myeloma, lymphoma, Hodgkin disease, and neuroblastoma.

The likelihood that an autologous transplant will succeed hinges on several factors. The patient must be healthy enough to withstand the rigors of a transplant. The disease must be sensitive to the particular combination of high-dose chemotherapy and/or radiation given prior to transplant. The transplant team must be skilled at spotting and managing complications that can arise from the treatment.

Although not all patients are cured by an autologous transplant, it may prolong and improve the quality of a patient's life for many years.

A Look Into the Future

There is considerable, promising research underway to improve upon the results now being achieved with autologous transplantation. Some investigators are testing new combinations of high-dose chemotherapy to determine which is most effective in destroying a particular disease. Others are investigating ways to make the patient's own immune system get rid of diseased cells that may remain after transplantation. Still others are exploring ways to prevent complications associated with the treatment.

Many people with diseases once thought incurable are now leading productive lives, thanks to progress made in the field of autologous transplantation.

Chapter Two
NUTS & BOLTS

I still find it bizarre that I would be the one to get so sick. I was very physically active. I rode my bike 2,000 miles a year, swam about 100 miles, and was active in my children's lives. Cancer happens to people you read about in the newspaper. It doesn't strike an enormously healthy, happy and vital 39-year-old family man.

Mike Eckhardt, 11-year transplant survivor

This chapter will give you a broad overview of autologous transplantation. The information can assist you in deciding whether or not to undergo a transplant, proceed with a decision you've already made, or understand the treatment that a loved one is undergoing. More detailed information about various aspects of autologous transplantation can be found in the remaining chapters of this book.

What are Bone Marrow and Stem Cells?

Bone marrow is a spongy tissue found inside bones. Bone marrow contains blood stem cells — special cells that generate most of the body's blood cells. Blood stem cells produce:

- white blood cells (leukocytes) to fight infection.

- red blood cells (erythrocytes) to carry oxygen to and remove waste products from organs and tissues.

- and platelets, which enable blood to clot.

If you are considering an autologous transplant, you may want to familiarize yourself with the different types of blood cells and their functions. During your treatment, the medical team will count and refer to these different blood cells frequently. (For a detailed discussion of blood cells, go to Appendix A, About Blood Cells, at the back of the book.)

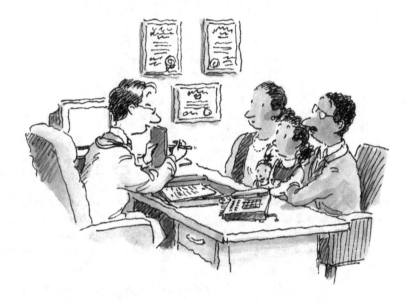

Why an Autologous Transplant?

Sometimes a patient cannot be cured of his disease with standard dosages of chemotherapy or radiation. A higher dosage of chemotherapy and/or radiation may cure the patient, but will also destroy the stem cells that create his blood cells. Without blood cells, the body cannot fight infection, get oxygen to tissues or allow blood to clot.

An autologous transplant lets doctors "rescue" a patient from the life threatening side effects of high-dose chemotherapy/radiation therapy. Stem cells are collected from the patient's bone marrow or bloodstream before the high-dose chemotherapy and/or radiation, and are returned to him after treatment. An autologous stem cell transplant is sometimes called an autologous stem cell rescue.

Source of Stem Cells

The earliest autologous transplants were autologous bone marrow transplants. Bone marrow is rich in the stem cells that produce the various types of blood cells.

In the mid-1980s, researchers discovered that stem cells could be moved out of the bone marrow into the bloodstream where they could be collected and used successfully in an autologous transplant. Stem cells collected from the bloodstream are called peripheral blood stem cells.

Who Can Undergo Autologous Transplantation?

To be a candidate for an autologous transplant, you must be healthy enough to tolerate the transplant procedure. Age, general physical condition, diagnosis and the stage of the disease are all considered by the physician when determining whether you are a good candidate for an autologous transplant.

Tests of your heart, lungs, kidneys and other vital organs are performed prior to transplant to ensure you can tolerate the procedure. If a tumor is present, its status will be evaluated at this time. The tests for organ function and tumor status are later used as a baseline against which post-transplant tests can be compared. The pre-transplant tests are usually done on an outpatient basis.

Stem Cell Harvest

Prior to the high-dose chemotherapy and/or radiation, your blood stem cells are collected. If the stem cells are collected from the bloodstream, the procedure is called a peripheral blood stem cell harvest. A stem cell harvest is usually performed in the outpatient clinic and is not a surgical procedure.

Prior to the harvest, a device called an apheresis catheter (a long flexible tube) is inserted into a large vein in the chest. This procedure is typically done with local anesthesia. The catheter makes it possible to collect stem cells without inserting needles into your hands or arms. Later, the catheter will be used to give you chemotherapy, other drugs and fluids, and to withdraw blood samples painlessly.

You will receive daily injections of a drug such as Neupogen® (filgrastim) or Mozobil® (plerixafor) which moves stem cells out of the bone marrow into the bloodstream where they are collected. Typically it takes one to three days to collect enough stem cells for transplant. Some patients also receive a small dosage of chemotherapy before the harvest to help move stem cells into the bloodstream and to shrink their tumor.

During the harvest, which can last two to six hours, you will sit in a comfortable chair. Blood will be withdrawn through the catheter and passed through flexible tubing to a machine called an apheresis machine, which separates out the stem cells and returns the rest of the blood to you. The stem cells are then cryopreserved (frozen at very low temperatures) until the day of transplant. It can take one to five days to collect enough stem cells for transplantation.

Some patients feel light headed, cold or numb around the lips during the collection. Others experience cramping in their hands caused by a blood-thinning agent used during the procedure that reduces the level of calcium in the blood. The cramping usually resolves after treatment with calcium supplements. Other possible short-term side effects include bone pain, headache, fatigue and nausea.

Bone Marrow Harvest

Some patients undergo a bone marrow harvest instead of a stem cell harvest. Occasionally, a patient may need to undergo both in order to collect sufficient stem cells for transplantation.

A bone marrow harvest is a surgical procedure that takes place in a hospital operating room. It involves minimal discomfort and little risk. While the patient is under anesthesia, a needle is inserted into the rear hip bone where a large quantity of bone marrow is located. The bone marrow, a thick red liquid, is extracted with a needle and syringe. The harvested bone marrow is then cryopreserved until the day of transplant.

Several skin punctures on each hip and multiple bone punctures are required to extract sufficient bone marrow for transplantation. There are no surgical incisions or stitches involved, only skin punctures where the needle is inserted.

The amount of bone marrow harvested depends on the size of the patient and the concentration of stem cells in the marrow. Usually, one to two quarts of marrow and blood are harvested. While this may sound like a lot, the body can usually replace it in four weeks.

When the anesthesia wears off, you may feel some discomfort at the harvest site. The pain will be similar to that associated with a hard fall on the ice and can usually be controlled with acetaminophen (Tylenol®). Patients can typically resume normal activities in a few days, although activities like climbing stairs or sitting in one place for a long period of time may be uncomfortable for a week or so.

Purging & CD34+ Selection

After the harvest, some centers process the stem cells to reduce the number of cancer cells in the sample. One of two techniques is used for this purpose: purging or CD34+ selection.

Purging is a process that uses either monoclonal antibodies or chemicals to kill cancer cells. Monoclonal antibodies are special proteins that can distinguish tumor cells from normal cells. When mixed with harvested stem cells, they attach themselves to tumor cells in the sample. Other proteins called "complement" or "immunotoxins" then find the "marked" cells and destroy them.

Alternatively, the stem cells may be incubated with chemicals that are more toxic to tumor cells than stem cells. This type of purging is called pharmacological purging.

CD34+ selection works on a different principle. Stem cells have a special marker on their surface called the CD34 antigen. Some tumor cells do not have this antigen on their surface. By passing the stem cell sample through a device called a cell separator, doctors can capture or "select" the cells with the CD34 antigen on magnetic beads or gels, and wash away the remaining cells in the sample.

A downside of purging and CD34+ selection is that some of the healthy stem cells are lost or destroyed during the process. If too few stem cells are transplanted into a patient, it may take longer for the your body to begin producing healthy new blood cells. It may also reduce the amount of bone marrow in the body after you recover from the transplant. This is a significant problem if the you relapse and need additional chemotherapy. Although most patients do not experience these problems, many centers reserve a portion of the harvested stem cells before purging or CD34+ selection. If the processed stem cells do not produce normal numbers of blood cells after transplantation, the reserved cells may be used to relieve the problem.

Preparative Regimen

After the stem cell or bone marrow harvest, you will undergo several days of chemotherapy and/or radiation to destroy the disease. This is called the preparative or conditioning regimen. The exact combination and dosage of chemotherapy and/or radiation varies according to the disease being treated and the protocol, or preferred treatment plan of the transplant facility. The preparative regimen usually lasts between four and ten days. (For more on this topic, see Chapter Seven, Preparative Regimen.)

The Transplant

One to three days after the preparative regimen, the transplant occurs. The stem cells collected from the bloodstream or bone marrow will be infused into you through the apheresis catheter. This procedure typically takes 30 minutes to an hour.

You will be awake and may be lightly sedated during the transplant. You will be checked frequently for signs of fever, chills, hives and chest pains. When the transplant is done, the days and weeks of waiting begin.

Engraftment

The two to three week period after the transplant is a critical time. The preparative regimen will have destroyed your stem cells, temporarily crippling your immune system. Until the transplanted stem cells migrate to the cavities of the bones and begin producing normal blood cells, you will be very susceptible to infection and excessive bleeding.

Drugs called growth factors may be given to speed recovery of blood counts. Multiple antibiotics and blood transfusions will be given to help prevent and fight infection. Platelet transfusions will help prevent bleeding.

Precautions will be taken to minimize exposure to viruses and bacteria. Medical personnel will wash their hands with antiseptic soap and may wear gloves and/or masks while visiting you. You may be required to wear a mask when you leave the clinic or their hospital room. The mask provides a barrier against bacteria and viruses, and reminds others that you are at high risk of developing an infection.

During this period, you may be instructed to avoid fresh vegetables, fruits, plants and cut flowers, since these items often carry bacteria that could cause a serious infection. You may also be told to avoid young children and certain pets until your immune system is functioning normally. (For more on infections see Chapter Eight, Infection.)

Daily blood samples are taken during this period to determine whether the stem cells have begun producing healthy blood cells. When blood counts begin to rise, the antibiotics and blood and platelet transfusions will generally no longer be required. Once the stem cells are producing a sufficient number of healthy blood cells, you will be discharged from the hospital or outpatient center, provided no other complications have developed.

Where Treatment is Given

Historically, patients were hospitalized during the preparative regimen, the transplant and the first few weeks of the recovery period. Now, many centers perform all or part of the treatment in an outpatient facility.

Patients treated in an outpatient facility typically spend four to twelve hours a day there during the preparative regimen and transplant. Following the transplant, patients visit the facility daily to receive blood and platelet transfusions, intravenous fluids, anti-nausea medications and antibiotics. At night, patients return home, to an apartment, or hotel room near the hospital where they are watched carefully by a family member or a friend who has been trained as their caregiver. (For more on caregivers, see Chapter Twelve, Caregiving.)

Some patients are hospitalized for all or part of their treatment. Hospitalization may be required if the patient does not have a caregiver to monitor him at home, or has medical problems that need around-the-clock monitoring by the medical staff.

How Patients Feel During Treatment

An autologous transplant is a physically and emotionally taxing procedure for both the patient and family. A patient should seek as much help as possible to cope with the transplant experience.

After the preparative regimen, patients often feel extremely tired, sick and weak. You may experience nausea, vomiting, fever and diarrhea. Activities like walking, sitting up in bed for long periods of time, reading books, talking on the phone, visiting with friends or even watching TV may require more energy than you have available.

Complications such as infection or bleeding can develop after transplant, creating additional discomfort. Mouth sores may make eating and swallowing uncomfortable.

Temporary mental confusion, usually related to the medications, sometimes occurs. This can be quite frightening for you and your family members who may not realize that it's temporary. The medical staff can help you deal with these problems.

Handling Emotional Stress

In addition to the physical discomfort, there's also emotional and psychological discomfort. Some patients find the emotional and psychological stress more problematic than the physical discomfort. They must not only handle the fact that they have a life-threatening disease, but many are fearful of the transplant procedure itself. While the transplant offers the hope of a cure or longer life, there are no guarantees. Living with that uncertainty can be very difficult.

Transplant patients can also feel quite isolated. Special precautions taken to guard against infection during recovery sometimes interfere with your ability to interact normally with family and friends. Some friends and family members may not understand, or be poorly equipped to manage the gravity of the situation and the emotional trauma involved in a transplant.

Helplessness is a common feeling among transplant patients, and can cause anger or resentment. For many, it is unnerving to be totally dependent on strangers for survival, no matter how competent they may be. Some also find it embarrassing to be dependent on others for help with basic daily functions such as using the washroom. Patients' unfamiliarly with the medical jargon used to describe the transplant procedure can make the feeling of helplessness worse.

The time spent waiting for blood counts to return to safe levels increases the emotional load. Recovery can be like a roller coaster ride: one day you may feel much better only to awake the next day feeling as sick as ever. (For more on the psychological and emotional aspects of an autologous transplant see Chapter Five, Emotional Challenges.)

First Year After Transplant

The length and nature of the recovery period varies from patient to patient. It may take six or more months before you are well enough to resume a normal routine and return to school or work. It is best not to set unrealistic recovery goals or compare your progress to another's. The length of the recovery period is not a good indication of whether or not you have been cured, or how long life has been extended. Some patients simply take longer to recover than others, and can look forward to a long, healthy life.

Sometimes transplant survivors develop an infection or other complication several weeks or months after transplant. If this happens to you, you may need to be hospitalized for treatment. This can be depressing, since you may be very anxious to put hospital routines behind you. It helps to keep in mind that these setbacks are common, and are usually temporary and reversible.

Life during the first year after transplant can be both exhilarating and worrisome. On the one hand, it is exciting to be alive after being so close to death. Many survivors find their quality of life improves after transplant.

Nonetheless, most worry that the disease will come back. It can be many months before a survivor has one full day pass without thinking about the disease or transplant experience. (For a discussion of long-term survival issues see Chapter Fifteen, Planning for Survivorship.)

Is It Worth It?

Many survivors who have been surveyed report that their quality of life after transplant is as good as or better than before. While autologous stem cell or bone marrow transplants are not always successful, they have cured or prolonged the lives of thousands of people. These survivors are grateful to have been given a new lease on life.

> "Currently, I'm 14-months post-transplant. I celebrated my one-year anniversary by climbing a mountain in Colorado and getting second row seats for a Jimmy Buffet concert. Lots of people celebrated with me and gave me inspirational messages, gifts and support. My favorite gift was from my doctor — an interpretation of my bone marrow biopsy. The interpretation pretty much describes my life today. Normal."

To learn more visit our web site at:

www.bmtinfonet.org/before/basics

Chapter Three
CHOOSING A TRANSPLANT CENTER

Was I scared? I was scared as a rabbit in winter. But I kept thinking, 'there's light at the end of the tunnel and I'm not ready to give up'. I remember the day they put me in the hospital. My 13-year-old son said 'I'm wrapping an invisible rope around you, Mom. Slowly but surely I'm going to tug on it until I get you back home again'. That was the most wonderful thing in the world. I'll never forget that he said that.

Maralyn Collins, 19-year transplant survivor

In the early days of transplantation, autologous transplants were offered by only a handful of medical centers worldwide. Today more than 200 centers perform autologous transplants in the U.S. alone. How do you decide which medical center is best for you?

Depending on your insurance coverage, the choice may be wide open or very limited. In the U.S., many insurers negotiate contracts with a handful of transplant centers and require their plan enrollees to be treated at these centers. Although such plans limit the patient's choices, the designated medical centers are usually major institutions with a highly experienced transplant team that provides excellent care.

Your particular disease may also limit the number of centers available for consideration. For example, while many centers perform autologous transplants for lymphoma and multiple myeloma, fewer offer transplants for diseases such as amyloidosis.

Your oncologist or hematologist may recommend a particular center based on a number of obvious factors, like the transplant team's experience and reputation. Other less obvious factors may include the relationship your doctor has with physicians at a particular center, and his prior experience in getting help and information from the center when the patient is returned to him for follow-up care. Ask why your doctor recommends one center over another, and don't hesitate to ask his opinion about other transplant centers as well.

BMT InfoNet maintains a list of centers that perform autologous transplants in the U.S. and Canada that includes information on the number of transplants performed, diseases treated, accreditation and contact information. You can access the list online at www.bmtinfonet.org/transplantcenters or by phoning 888-597-7674.

If you are free to choose between different centers, there are several factors you'll want to consider. The rest of this chapter will explore some of these issues and provide guidance on how to find the center that's right for you.

Accreditation

The Foundation for Accreditation of Cellular Therapy (FACT) is an organization that inspects transplant programs and accredits those that meet the FACT standards. Although transplant centers are not required to seek FACT accreditation, FACT accreditation is a sign that the program has passed a rigorous inspection and is considered by experts in the field to be a quality transplant program.

Go to www.factwebsite.org to learn which programs are FACT accredited.

The Transplant Team

When considering a transplant center, focus first on the transplant team — the doctors, nurses, radiologists, pharmacists and other support staff who will be involved in your care. The more training and experience they have in dealing with transplant patients, the better able they'll be to respond to problems. Ask not only about the training and experience of individual team members, but how long they have been working together as a team.

Doctors

FACT standards require that the transplant program director be a licensed physician with board certification in hematology, medical oncology, immunology and/or pediatric hematology/oncology. Some physicians who completed their medical training before 1985 may not be board certified in one of these specialties, but may nonetheless have many years of experience in the field of autologous transplantation. Such doctors should be able to provide you with a list of publications they've authored that demonstrate their experience.

The other transplant physicians who will be involved in your care should also be licensed and board certified in one of the specialties described above.

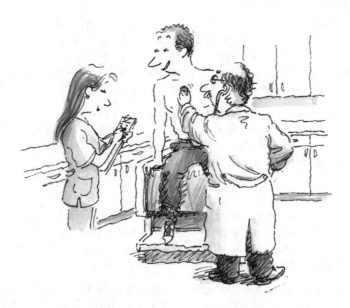

Ask if they've had extensive training or experience in the care of transplant patients. Will a *transplant* physician be on call 24-hours a day to handle emergencies and answer questions? If you have a pre-existing medical condition that may complicate your treatment, such as heart or lung problems, ask specifically about the doctors' experience in handling patients with similar problems.

Be sure the transplant team has around-the-clock access to other licensed specialists who may need to be involved in your care. This includes doctors who are board certified in surgery, pulmonary medicine, intensive care, gastroenterology, nephrology, infectious diseases, cardiology, pathology, psychiatry and radiation therapy.

Nurses

A highly-trained, experienced team of nurses is a critical component of a good transplant program. It's the nurses who spend the most time with patients. They must be able to quickly identify problems and respond appropriately.

Find out how many registered nurses will be involved in your care. How many have been trained and certified in hematology/oncology? How much experience have they had caring for autologous transplant patients? Ask about the nurse-to-patient ratio, and any ongoing education the nurses receive.

Psychosocial Support Services

Undergoing an autologous transplant is not only physically difficult, but emotionally taxing as well. Some patients find the emotional trauma more difficult to handle than the physical discomfort. People who have never before sought psychiatric counseling may need the help of a psychiatrist, psychologist, social worker, or religious counselor to help them cope with the transplant experience.

Psychosocial support services offered by transplant centers vary considerably. Ask whether psychiatric help is routinely provided to patients or is available upon request. Find out what other programs are available to help patients and family members cope with the emotional stress.

Pediatric Patients

If the transplant patient is a child, find out whether the doctors, nurses and support staff have training and experience in treating pediatric patients. Children are not just small adults. Their growing bodies may react differently to drugs, and their emotional needs are different as well.

Some transplant centers specialize in treating only pediatric patients, while others treat both children and adults — sometimes with the same staff. If the center you're considering does not limit its practice to pediatric patients, be sure that the team members, as well as consulting specialists, are experienced in caring for pediatric patients.

Some centers have strict guidelines about how long the parent can remain with a hospitalized child and require parents to leave in the evening. Others will allow parents to remain overnight if they wish. Make sure you're comfortable with the center's guidelines on this matter.

Ask what sort of age-appropriate activities and counseling will be provided to your child during her treatment. Inquire about the center's philosophy on providing pain medications before, during and after painful procedures such as bone marrow aspirates. Can your child bring favorite toys, clothes, etc. with her to the hospital room? Rules vary considerably at different centers on these matters, and you should be sure you're comfortable with their approach before your child is admitted. (For more on pediatric transplant issues see Chapter Six, When Your Child Needs a Transplant.)

Support For Caregivers

Many transplant programs now provide some or all of the treatment in the outpatient clinic. This means that a primary caregiver must be available to monitor and care for the patient when he returns home.

Ask what sort of support systems are in place to help caregivers. Find out what kind of training caregivers will receive, and whether the caregiver will have access to volunteers who can help with routine daily tasks while the caregiver is with the patient, particularly if the transplant is taking place out of town.

Number of Transplants Performed

Although the training and experience of the transplant team members are the most important factors to evaluate, the number of transplants performed by a center can often give you a rough idea of the team's experience. Keep in mind, however, that transplant teams and team members frequently relocate to different hospitals. Fifty transplants may have been performed at a center during the past two years, but not necessarily by the team that will care for you now.

You can find out how may transplants have been preformed at a center by inquiring at the center directly, by contacting BMT InfoNet at 888-597-7674 or online at www.bmtinfonet.org/transplantcenters.

Treatment Plans

The treatment plan or "protocol" for a particular disease can vary from center to center. The type and dosage of chemotherapy drugs may differ. Some centers may be testing new methods of handling transplant complications. Others may be investigating novel ways to prevent relapse.

The risks associated with various treatment plans may differ as well. Ask what is known about the effectiveness and risks associated with the particular protocol suggested for you. Find out what will be done to manage the complications, and satisfy yourself that the center has the experience necessary to spot and quickly treat problems when they arise.

You might want to ask how many patients have already undergone the same treatment at that particular center, how many have developed problems, and how many have benefitted from the treatment. Ask the doctor to be as specific as possible in describing how patients that are similar to you (e.g., same age, stage of disease and medical problems) have fared. Keep in mind, however, that such data may not be available for newer treatment plans.

Success Rates

The question asked most often by patients is "Which transplant center has the best success rate?" Success rates quoted by centers can be very misleading if not properly interpreted.

A "successful transplant" can be defined in different ways. It may mean that the stem cells engrafted and the patient did not die of complications while in the hospital or clinic. Alternatively, "successful transplant" may mean that the patient lived one, three, five years or more without a recurrence of the disease. When discussing success rates with transplant centers, be sure you understand how they are defining the term.

Transplant teams may use the terms "event-free survival" (EFS) or "disease-free survival" (DFS) when discussing their success rate. Although they sound similar, each statistic measures success differently.

Event-free survival tells you how many patients, out of all that were transplanted, are alive and disease-free a specific number of years after transplant. If 100 patients were transplanted for Hodgkin disease and 40 are still alive and disease-free three years after transplant, the three year event-free survival is 40 percent.

Disease-free survival, on the other hand, focuses only on the patients who were *in remission* after transplant. In other words, if only 50 out of 100 patients were in remission after their transplant, and forty were alive and disease-free three years after transplant, the three year disease-free survival rate will be 80 percent (40 patients divided by 50).

On first glance it might look like the transplant center with the 80 percent disease-free survival had more successful transplants than the center with 40 percent event-free survival but, in fact, their success rates are similar. Both had 40 of 100 patients alive and disease free after transplant.

Don't compare event-free survival rates at one center to disease-free survival rates at another. It's like comparing apples to oranges. Ask for both figures, and be sure they are for a comparable group of patients followed over a comparable length of time.

Many factors influence a center's success rate. For example, a hospital that accepts only prime candidates for transplant — young persons, those in an early stage of their disease, and those who have responded well to prior treatment — may report better success rates than centers who treat older or sicker patients.

When asking about success rates, be sure the figure you're given pertains to treatment at that particular center, using the same protocol and for the same disease. Success rates for patients who were treated with a different protocol may not be a good gauge of how well you'll fare with the treatment plan proposed for you. Success rates from other centers may be better or worse than success rates achievable at the center you're considering.

Finances

Autologous transplants are very costly, even if insurance is paying for all or most of the procedure. In addition to medical expenses, families may incur large travel, lodging and meal expenses, particularly if the patient is being treated out of town. If a caregiver must take time off from work to be with the patient, this can add to the financial burden.

Additional child care expenditures may be necessary while a parent is being treated. Incidental expenses such as phone calls, purchases of snacks and gifts and parking fees can add up, particularly if the patient must be hospitalized for a lengthy period of time.

Talk to the social worker at the transplant center to find out what sort of assistance is available to help defray these expenses. Some centers have special arrangements with local hotels or dormitories to house patients and family members at low or no cost. Others can help you apply for financial assistance.

If convincing your insurance company to pay for the transplant is a problem, find out what sort of help the center will provide. Some are well prepared to handle insurance company inquiries and are experienced in persuading insurers to pay for your care. Others are not. Ask how successful the center has been in helping appeal an insurer's denial of coverage should that occur. (For more on insurance problems see Chapter Four, Insurance and Fundraising.)

If insurance refuses to pay for your treatment, ask what sort of alternative financing arrangements the center is willing to make with you. Most centers will refuse to provide treatment unless insurance pre-approves payment or the family makes a hefty down payment.

Charges for autologous transplants vary considerably from center to center. A center may not be able to quote an exact price for your treatment, since the cost of your care will depend on whether or not you need to be hospitalized and any special treatment needs. Do, however, ask for a ballpark estimate of the cost, particularly if you are going to have to pay for the treatment.

Long-Term Follow-Up

After you leave the center, your care will eventually be turned over to your local doctor, ideally a specialist like an oncologist or hematologist. Since most doctors have not received specific training in the care of transplant patients, it's important that the transplant center staff be accessible to both you and your doctor to handle questions and provide guidance about your care. Many transplant centers strongly encourage patients to return to the center annually, at least for the first few years, for follow-up care.

Find out whether the transplant center will keep your own doctor updated on your treatment and progress. Ask if you and your doctor will receive written instructions about follow-up care. Both you and your doctor should feel comfortable contacting your transplant center directly to discuss questions and concerns.

Guidelines for long-term follow-up care of autologous transplant patients have been developed by the American Society of Blood and Marrow Transplantation, the Center for International Blood and Marrow Transplant Research and The European Group for Blood & Marrow Transplantation. You can access these guidelines through the BMT InfoNet web site at www.bmtinfonet.org/after/protecthealthlongterm or by phoning 888-597-7674.

The Bottom Line

Happily, there are many excellent transplant programs that provide top-quality medical care. For most patients, no one program will clearly be superior. Rather, you and your doctor will be able to choose among a number of excellent, highly qualified transplant programs.

Keep in mind that you and your family are important members of the transplant team. It's important that you're comfortable with the staff at the center where you'll be treated, and that worries about issues such as insurance, and having family members close at hand or well cared for, are kept to a minimum. Working with your doctor, you should be able to identify the programs that best suit your family's medical, financial and emotional needs.

To learn more go to our web site at:

www.bmtinfonet.org/before/choosingtransplantcenter

Chapter Four
INSURANCE AND FUNDRAISING

Our insurance company said a transplant was experimental and would not approve it. During an unbelievably stressful week, we contacted an attorney, looked into private pay options and asked the hospital how they could help. I don't know whether it was the letters from our transplant center and our attorney, or calls from us and my employer that did it, but a week later they changed their mind and agreed to pay for the transplant.

Julie Brodeur, mother of Amanda Brodeur, five-year transplant survivor

Most transplant centers are skilled at providing insurers with the documentation they need to authorize coverage of an autologous transplant. Fortunately, many patients have no difficulty persuading their insurer to pay for their treatment.

However, if you have difficulty with your insurance company, read on. The information in this section will help you understand how insurance companies make decisions, how you can appeal those decisions, when to enlist the help of an experienced attorney and what other funding options exist.

Insurance

An autologous transplant is a very expensive medical procedure. Depending on the transplant center, the length of time you must be hospitalized, and complications that arise, the treatment can cost hundreds of thousands of dollars. It's therefore not surprising that some insurance providers balk at paying for this treatment.

The best way to minimize insurance problems is to start early. Since life gets more hectic if an insurance denial comes at the last minute, it's important that you and the transplant center take a few steps at the outset.

Plan Ahead

As soon as possible, ask the insurer to pre-approve the treatment. The transplant center, not you, should contact your insurer early in the planning process so that the company can review the request and resolve questions.

The transplant center should set a target date for starting your treatment and communicate that date to the insurer when they seek pre-approval. This gives the insurer a deadline by which it must decide whether or not to pay for the treatment. If a patient has to go to court in order to get an insurer to cover the treatment, it's easier if an optimum transplant time has been determined in advance, say attorneys experienced in this field.

It's also wise to gather all your insurance information early on. Get the latest copy of your full plan booklet (not the summary booklet usually given to plan participants), as well as copies of any other policies under which you are insured (any secondary policies). If you later need to consult with an attorney, she will need all these documents to determine whether the insurer is legally required to cover the treatment under the terms of the contract.

Submit Complete Information

Many transplant centers send an information package to the insurer that includes a letter from the treating physician, as well as studies and articles supporting the recommended procedure. It's important that insurers get this information early on, and that it be complete and up-to-date. The letter from the doctor should stress that the treatment is the best available therapy for the patient, is safe and effective, and is widely accepted by the medical community. Articles and letters of support that explain why the treatment plan is appropriate should be current.

If Coverage is Denied

If your insurance company denies coverage of your medical treatment, don't take "no" for an answer. It's often possible to reverse that decision.

Usually when insurers deny coverage for an autologous transplant, they rely on language in the insurance contract that excludes payment for experimental or investigational treatments. What insurers or physicians may consider experimental, however, can be quite different from the legal definition of experimental.

It's wise to consult an attorney who is experienced in this field of law to determine whether or not you may be able to successfully reverse a denial of coverage. Your letter of appeal should *not* be drafted by the attorney who helped you with your house closing or divorce. You need an attorney who is just as experienced in this field of law as your doctor is in this field of medicine.

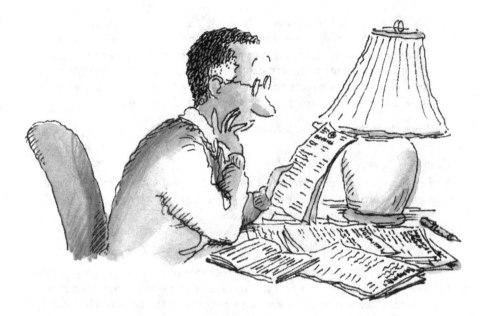

Your transplant center may have the name of an attorney who successfully helped patients in the past. If not, you can contact BMT InfoNet at 888-597-7674 for a referral to an attorney who can help you.

Appealing a Denial of Coverage

The majority of insurance plans are governed by ERISA, a federal law that requires you to do certain things within certain time frames if insurance coverage is denied. In most cases, you must first appeal your denial of coverage with the insurer before proceeding to a court appeal.

What you put in the letter of appeal will determine your rights later on, should you have to go to court. Accordingly, you should keep the following points in mind.

1. In most cases, you are required to appeal a denial of coverage within 60 days or you lose all further rights of appeal. Some people are turned down at the last moment and go forward with treatment, figuring they'll deal with the insurance problem later on. When they do get around to filing an appeal, it may be too late.

2. You and your doctor should include *all* evidence supporting the appropriateness of the therapy when you file the appeal. In most cases, if you later have to go to court to appeal an insurer's denial of coverage, the issue will be whether or not the insurer made an appropriate decision in light of the evidence it received from your doctor. If important studies or other evidence are omitted from your letter of appeal, you may not be able to offer them as evidence at a later trial.

3. The appeal letter should clearly state why the procedure is appropriate for the treatment of your disease. It should identify all resources the insurer should contact, list any favorable second opinions you received, and include instructions on how to contact doctors rendering these favorable opinions. Some transplant centers include in their appeal packet several letters from respected doctors who endorse the treatment.

4. Keep the letter professional and friendly.

Going to Court

If an insurance company turns down a letter of appeal and you haven't already consulted an attorney, it's important that you do so immediately. Some patients erroneously believe that involving an attorney in the dispute will result in delay and jeopardize their chance to receive treatment in a timely manner. In fact, the reverse is usually true.

An experienced attorney can determine whether you have good legal grounds to challenge the denial of coverage. Often it takes little more than a letter from an attorney to the insurance company to cause the company to reconsider its opinion. If negotiations fail, an attorney may seek a temporary restraining order.

It typically takes a matter of days to obtain a temporary restraining order. If granted, patients can proceed with the treatment and the insurance company is required to pay for the treatment until a full court trial takes place and a final decision is rendered.

Often, if a judge issues a temporary restraining order, the insurer will reach a settlement with the patient, rather than proceed to a full court trial. Trials are costly and insurers often prefer to settle rather than risk an adverse legal decision that will set a precedent for future cases.

In the event that insurance does not cover some or all of a transplant and it becomes necessary to secure funding elsewhere, there are several options to consider.

Life Insurance, Viatical Settlements and Accelerated Benefits

Life insurance was once considered a source of funds only after a person died. But policies are changing, sometimes to the benefit of the policyholder. Two options have become popular for owners of life insurance who are terminally or chronically ill — viatical settlements and accelerated benefits. Both provide cash benefits while the policyholder is still alive. These benefits may be wholly or partially exempt from federal taxes, thanks to the enactment of the Health Insurance Portability and Accountability Act.

Viatical Settlements

Viatical settlements appeared in the 1980s in reaction to the AIDS crisis. Brokers offered to purchase life insurance policies at a discount from terminally ill patients. They would then sell them to a viatical settlement provider who made a cash payment to the patient. Patients were free to use the money for medical expenses, or any other purpose.

Soon an industry arose with good and bad results. Patients who truly needed cash had a new source of funds. However, some received far less than the true value of their policy.

To ensure that vulnerable patients are protected, many states now require viatical settlement providers to be licensed. The National Association of Insurance Commissioners (NAIC) has adopted the Viatical Settlements Model Act as a guideline for reasonable payments.

In order for the proceeds from a viatical settlement to be exempt from federal taxes, the viatical settlement provider must either be licensed by the state or meet the model guidelines of the NAIC.

Accelerated Benefits

Some life insurance policies have an accelerated benefits option. Many older group life plans do not contain a specific provision providing for accelerated benefits, but may offer it as an exception on a case-by-case basis.

Many plans offer up to 75 percent of your benefit now, with the balance reserved as a true death benefit. There is usually an interest or transaction fee charged for taking an accelerated benefit.

The advantages of taking accelerated benefits rather than selling a policy to a viatical settlement provider are two-fold: it is often less costly to take accelerated benefits, and you have the advantage of working with someone you know and trust. A disadvantage is that the insurance company may restrict the amount of benefits you can accelerate or put restrictions on how you use the funds.

Is It Right for Me?

If you are considering a viatical settlement or accelerating your life insurance benefits, the following points should be considered:

1. Is there really a need for the money?

    Funds you withdraw now will not be available to pay for expenses they were originally intended to cover such as education and living expenses of your survivors. Do you really need the funds? Funding normal living expenses and some small last luxuries makes sense for almost everyone. But there have been cases where people received viatical settlements and went on spending sprees to the detriment of their families and creditors. Examine why you want the funds and consider other options for securing necessary cash.

2. How will a viatical settlement or receipt of accelerated benefits affect your overall financial picture?

    An infusion of cash from a viatical settlement or accelerated benefits may affect your entitlement to public benefits, treatment of estate taxes and how your creditors view you. Some creditors may look to your viatical settlement funds as a ready source of payment. They may be less willing to enter into payment plans, and may demand immediate payment.

    Check with a social worker or benefits counselor to determine the settlement's effect on benefits such as disability or Medicaid. Speak with your accountant or attorney to determine what the tax and estate consequences will be. Keep in mind that life insurance is generally not accessible by creditors and passes on to your estate. If you receive the money earlier, you and your heirs may lose control over those funds.

3. Does your insurance policy provide accelerated benefits?

    Before entering into a viatical settlement, check to see if your life insurance plan offers an accelerated benefits option. Accelerated benefits can be cheaper and easier than a viatical settlement because it is already part of your policy.

4. Get the best deal.

    Some viatical settlements offer the patient as little as 30 percent of the total life insurance proceeds. On a $300,000 life insurance policy, that would be $90,000 to you and $210,000 to the settlement provider. The amount is often dependent on life expectancy. Shop around for the best deal, and be sure the provider is licensed by your state or conforms to the NAIC model guidelines.

Other Fundraising Options

A number of organizations provide financial support for some of the costs associated with transplants. Others will help patients and families conduct fundraisers. For a listing of these organizations, visit our online Resource Directory at www.bmtinfonet.org/resources or phone 888-597-7674.

To learn more go to our web site at:

www.bmtinfonet.org/before/financesinsurance

Chapter Five
EMOTIONAL CHALLENGES

There weren't any support groups for transplant patients in my area. If there had been a support group, I would have attended, because when they first tell you about the transplant and you start reading up on the subject, it can scare the heck out of you.

Dwight Gambral, 13-year transplant survivor

Autologous transplantation provides hope for many patients diagnosed with diseases that were once thought incurable. This hope sustains patients and their families through the difficult period of treatment and recovery. Nonetheless, contemplating an autologous transplant, undergoing the procedure and coping with the recovery process is a trying experience for patients, families and friends.

This chapter will discuss the fears and emotions that are typical during transplant. Throughout the chapter you will find direct quotations from persons who survived their transplant and have offered to share their insights.

Coping With the News

When a patient faces the prospect of an autologous transplant, the news can be devastating. Many will not yet have come to grips with the fact that they're suffering from a life-threatening disease. Deciding whether or not to undergo an autologous transplant increases the emotional turmoil. Sometimes the decision must be made quickly to provide the greatest likelihood of success, adding more stress to an already difficult situation.

The sheer volume of information can be overwhelming. Patients' lack of familiarity with medical jargon can make it difficult to understand doctors' explanations. Some simply cannot absorb new information while they are still struggling with so many other details about their disease. Patients may ask the same question repeatedly, failing each time to understand the answer.

Little of the information patients receive will sound like good news. What patients want to hear is that the transplant will be a quick, painless, risk-free procedure. More importantly, they want assurance that it will cure their disease and provide them with many extra years of life. Unfortunately, no such assurances can be given. The patient can only be promised the chance of a future.

Fear that more unsettling news is forthcoming precludes many patients from asking questions. As much as they may want answers, some opt to cope with uncertainty rather than open themselves up to more disturbing information.

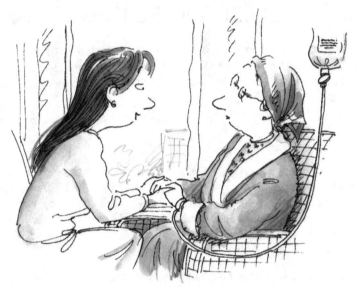

Getting Information

Doctors strive hard to give patients a complete and honest description of the transplant experience. They want patients to be fully informed about possible risks before undergoing the procedure. In doing so, however, doctors some-time confuse and overwhelm patients. They may assume that patients are familiar with medical terms like catheters, i.v., aspirates and biopsies. Often that is not the case. As one patient put it, "doctors talk medical, patients talk human".

Don't be embarrassed to ask your doctor to repeat something or to translate it into words that you can understand. Sometimes, asking one of the nurses to explain what the doctor means will help you better understand the message. Keep asking questions until you're satisfied with the answer, regardless of how many repetitions it takes.

It helps to write down any questions you have before visiting with your doctor. Some patients find that tape recording or videotaping their initial discussion with the transplant team helps answer questions that later arise. Others find that keeping an ongoing file with brochures, handouts, personal notes, and resource information can be useful to refer to throughout the process.

> "Your mind is going to explode with all the things you have to remember or want to ask. Write down the questions you want to ask as well as the doctors' answers to your questions. If you don't get a straight answer or don't understand the answer, ask again until it is clear."

> "It's important to make sure that the doctor talks with you about the items on *your* agenda, not just his. You need to be assertive. My 23-year-old daughter, for example, wanted to talk about infertility and options for having a child after the transplant. The doctors wanted to brush that issue aside."

Family and friends can help you sort through the deluge of information received from a doctor. If you are afraid or embarrassed to ask a physician the same question for the tenth time, you will appreciate a family member who can ask the question on your behalf.

Putting Things Into Perspective

For many patients, the list of possible complications is frightening and overwhelming. Ask your doctor to help you put them into perspective. Don't assume that the risk of death or severe liver damage, for example, is as great as the risk of temporary hair loss or mouth sores. (It's not!)

Some patients find it helpful to group the possible complications into three categories: those that will definitely occur, those that often occur and those that rarely occur. In doing this, the risk is put into perspective and can ease your worries.

Doctors sometimes forget to mention that pain relief will be provided when needed. Thus, when patients hear about the numerous complications that might occur, they assume they'll be in terrible pain. While there may be some painful complications associated with the transplant, there are a variety of effective pain medications available. (For more about pain see Chapter Eleven, Relieving Pain.)

Setting Goals

The time spent preparing for, undergoing and recovering from an autologous transplant can seem never-ending. Patients seldom make daily progress by leaps and bounds. Each day will bring a small step forward, maybe a little backsliding, or no change at all. This slow pace of progress can discourage patients (and their loved ones) who want desperately to get well and put this chapter of their life behind them.

Ask the doctors and nurses to help you set realistic goals, and to tell you each time progress is made, no matter how small. Patients constantly feel overwhelmed by bad news. Any progress or positive news, no matter how small, can buoy your spirits.

> "Progress can be so very slow. I found it was helpful to keep charts so that I could see that progress was being made. Drinking an ounce of water an hour adds up to a lot of fluid by the end of the day. Walking three feet today and increasing it by two feet each day is a lot by the end of the week."

It helps to take one day at a time rather than worry about what will happen in five days, five weeks or five years.

Encouraging comments from family members on days when a patient looks better can boost the patient's morale. On those days when setbacks occur, it's best for family members to discuss their disappointment with someone other than the patient.

Loss of Control

> "In the beginning, I was a very angry patient. I was very bitter and scared. Anger was my way of coping."

An autologous transplant is a physically debilitating experience. You will be in a fragile state of health for several weeks following the transplant, and will feel extremely weak and helpless. Walking without assistance, focusing on a book or television show, following the thread of a conversation, or even sitting up in bed may require more energy you have to spare.

Patients who are used to being in charge, taking care of themselves, or being the person upon whom others depend will find this physical debilitation discouraging. The loss of control can both frighten and anger a patient. His anger may be directed at physicians, other medical personnel or at loved ones.

It helps to assure the patient that a loved one will be his advocate while he is too weak to fend for himself. If a patient needs pain relief, has questions, or needs some other form of help, being able to rely on a loved one to track down the appropriate medical personnel and get the problem solved can be an immense relief. Patients know that the physicians and nurses are juggling the needs of many patients. Knowing that a loved one will advocate for them, and only them, can be very comforting.

Patients often react angrily to people who try to dictate rather than tactfully encourage them to do things they would rather not do. Giving the patient a chance to assert some control over his care can reduce feelings of helplessness and anger.

It's also important to respect the patient's modesty and privacy. As sick and helpless as the patient may be, there's no reason to require him to bare his body and soul to the world.

Patients often need time alone with physicians, psychologists, or social workers to discuss private concerns and feelings. Family members and friends should respect this need. Sitting in on discussions, especially between the patient and psychological or pastoral counselors, may prevent the patient from expressing feelings and concerns with which he needs help coping.

Isolation

The special precautions taken to protect a patient against infection while the immune system is recovering make many patients feel lonely and isolated. Transplant patients crave a normal environment where they're not the center of attention, where they can interact freely with family and friends, and where they can think about something other than their disease and treatment.

While the patient is hospitalized or staying in a facility away from home, decorating the room with things that are special to the patient can make him feel less detached from normal life. This can be done by having pictures of family members on hand, displaying cards and well wishes, and hanging pictures on the wall chosen by the patient. Bringing in the patient's own bed clothes, an MP3 player, books, a computer or a DVD player can also make the room seem homier.

When family and friends call or visit, they should talk about the world outside. Positive, upbeat anecdotes about family members and friends, descriptions of stores or museums visited, plays or movies that have been seen, the latest gossip from work or school — anything that brings the outside world to the patient — will make him feel less isolated and cut off from normal life.

Stressful Side Effects

Some side effects of the high-dose chemotherapy or radiation can be stressful for patients.

Temporary hair loss can change one's self image. It's common for a patient to feel self-conscious or embarrassed to be seen by family and friends. Wearing a head scarf, or hat can make a patient feel less conspicuous and, for some, is more comfortable than a wig.

Meals, too, can be stressful. Mouth sores, a common side effect of the treatment, can make eating uncomfortable. Some of the drugs administered to patients during treatment may temporarily alter the taste of foods. Providing patients with some of their favorite foods, and helping them find other foods that taste good can help lift the patient's spirits. (For more on eating difficulties see Chapter Ten, Nutrition.)

The large quantity of medications that patients need to take orally each day can be daunting, and some may have difficulty as they try to force down the pills. The tests administered to monitor the patient's overall physical condition, while not painful, can leave him feeling like his body is under constant assault. Though little can be done to curtail these necessary medications and tests, sympathy from all caregivers can help a patient cope.

In some cases, it is possible to reduce the physical discomfort associated with a procedure and thus reduce stress. Lightly sedating a patient prior to a bone marrow aspiration, for example, can make the procedure more comfortable. Do not be reluctant to ask for pre-medication or other pain relief if you're worried about discomfort.

Family members should take an active, aggressive role in advising physicians and nurses of the patient's discomfort and needs. Family members know the patient's personality best and will know the extent to which he will be stoic about pain and discomfort before asking for help. The medical team needs to know if he will request relief as soon as pain begins or only after the discomfort is really intense. The speed with which they respond to a patient's call for help is often influenced by this important information. (For more about pain relief see Chapter Eleven, Relieving Pain.)

Managing Anxiety

Anxiety and distress are a normal and expected part of the transplant experience. Patients who become very anxious or agitated are not weaklings or losing their minds. They're reacting in a very normal way to a very stressful experience.

> "During my transplant I was very depressed. My dad asked a co-worker, who had a transplant five years earlier, to visit me and share what he had been through. He said my feelings were acceptable, that he had been depressed, too, but now he's better and working full-time. I could look at him and see that he was a normal person. That helped me more than anything."

Many transplant patients benefit from the services of a psychiatrist, psychologist or social worker following diagnosis, during treatment and while recovering. If your physician does not volunteer these helpful services to you, ask for them.

Some patients are surprised or embarrassed that they are having trouble coping with the anxiety on their own. This is particularly true for people who have never before sought mental health services. Needing help coping with your emotions during treatment is normal. If you need counseling or the help of psychiatrist it does not mean that you are falling apart, or that you will require ongoing services after recovery.

"It's important to be honest with your own feelings. If you need help dealing with what you are about to face, seek it. This is not a sign of weakness. Sometimes, talking with someone who's been through the situation helps you separate, evaluate and move in a healthier direction."

Psychiatrists often help patients manage anxiety with sedatives and anti-depressant medications. Short-term use of these drugs by transplant patients is common, and does not lead to long-term drug dependency.

Insomnia

Sedatives and sleeping pills are particularly helpful in managing a problem experienced by many transplant patients — insomnia. Deprived of sleep, you can quickly become exhausted, unfocused and extremely irritable, making it even harder to cope with daytime stresses. Medications are available to counteract insomnia; there's no need to put up with sleepless nights and the stress they produce.

"Right before the transplant I had a lot of trouble sleeping. The whole thing was such a shock. Eventually a friend of mine who is a pediatrician suggested I get a prescription for sleeping pills. They really helped and they weren't addictive."

"I had trouble sleeping when going through my transplant, and still do sometimes. I found that active relaxation helps. Rather than laying awake, I get up and do some exercises — a few leg lifts or sit ups. It helps me relax and get back to sleep."

Keeping in Touch With Friends

Throughout much of the treatment and recovery period, the patient may be much too weak to visit with guests or even accept phone calls. Nonetheless, it's important for a patient to know that family members, friends, and co-workers are concerned about his progress and hoping for his recovery. It can be very depressing for a patient to feel that he has been forgotten by someone.

Cards and words of encouragement passed along through family members or friends can mean a lot to a patient who is feeling isolated.

"My family and friends put together an album for me when I was in the hospital, and everyone contributed something. There were pictures and all sorts of silly things — it was wonderful. Another friend, who is a professional photographer, gathered everyone in the park, took their picture and blew it up. I'm talking poster-size. It included everyone — my family, my friends, my coworkers — everyone. I loved it."

> "I arranged for my wife to hear messages left by well-wishers on the answering machine. It cheered her to know that so many people were thinking of her, and eliminated the problem of having the phone ring when she wasn't up to taking calls."

If you have access to the internet, services like CaringBridge.org or LotsaHelpingHands.org are a great way to keep in touch with family and friends. You can create a personal web page to post daily updates about the patient's progress for people to read. Visitors to your site can leave news about what's going on in their life as well as words of encouragement for the patient.

Sometimes people are afraid to intrude and therefore do not call or write. If you are a friend or family member who is concerned about intruding, check first with a close family member. More often than not your expression of concern will boost the patient's spirits.

Other gestures like donating platelets for the patient, helping with family household chores, caring for the patient's children, providing an evening off for the patient's support person, or filling in for the patient until she returns to work will also be greatly appreciated.

> "My co-workers cut my grass, brought meals and cleaned my house. During a heat wave, my church installed an air conditioner in my husband's room. Accepting this help was uplifting. I felt like I wasn't alone."

> "One thing that friends and co-workers did that did NOT help was tell me stories about people with cancer who didn't make it. I didn't really need to hear that and sometimes that can still set me off. Instead of saying, 'Please don't share any more with me,' or, 'I'd prefer not to hear this,' I'd just stand there and listen. That was stupid. In retrospect, I should have just politely cut it off."

During the recovery period, transplant patients want to feel normal and be treated as such. They don't want pity. They want to be able to take care of themselves to the extent possible, and don't want to be singled out for special treatment.

Family members, friends and co-workers sometimes have difficulty re-establishing a relationship with the survivor. Survivors will look different. They may have lost weight, be wearing a face mask to protect against infection, look physically drained, and have no hair. Because the patient will have been out of circulation for several weeks, he or she will not have shared as many experiences with family members or friends as usual. Visitors can feel awkward as they grope for an appropriate topic of conversation, and this awkwardness can discourage some people from calling or visiting.

"I had one friend who was so afraid to come near me that when she would visit, she'd drive up to the front of the house, beep her horn, wave to me and then drive off. That really hurt. Others would come right into my house, put on rubber gloves, help wash and feed me — they were wonderful. They will always be my dearest and closest friends."

In some cases, particularly with children, ignorance may make a person fearful of associating with the patient. One high school adolescent reported that, upon her return to school, the school corridors would literally clear out each time she appeared. The other teens were afraid they might "catch it" and were uncomfortable interacting with a classmate they believed was about to die.

Friends and family members of survivors can overcome some of this post-transplant awkwardness by not losing touch with the patient while he is undergoing treatment. Sharing normal life experiences with the patient either during a visit, by a note, or with a phone call can make re-establishing relationships after a transplant easier.

"My friend Roz was really great. She'd call and say, 'How are you?,' and then would start talking about all the things we used to talk about before the transplant. She wouldn't avoid the subject of the transplant, but she treated me just like she did before."

Children of adult transplant patients, as well as friends and classmates of children undergoing a transplant, should be prepared for the return of the patient, with the myths of catching it or the inevitability of the patient's death dispelled well in advance. This will not only ease the patient's stress, but also relieve unspoken fears the children may have about their parent or friend.

BMT Infonet offers a book for young children called *Mira's Month* that explains, with colorful pictures and age-appropriate language, what a child can expect when a parent undergoes a transplant. You can order the book online at www.bmtinfonet.org/products/book or by phoning 888-597-7674.

Oftentimes, friends will be unsure about how and when to re-establish a normal relationship with you, and will look for a cue from you before making a move. Some patients find that asking friends to help with a small task such as picking up a prescription at the drug store, taking their child to a school event, or returning a purchased item to a department store, will break the ice and let friends know that the survivor is ready for their companionship.

Friends can help ease the transition back to normal life by inviting patients to accompany them to places or events that do not pose undue health risks. Despite the fact that physical changes, such as hair loss, may make patients feel conspicuous, most will have a strong desire to get back into the normal flow of life, and the invitation will be much appreciated.

And Many Months Beyond

While memories of the transplant experience dim with time, the trauma will be remembered for a long time. It can take months before a survivor gets through a single day without reflecting on the transplant experience. Innocent remarks or events totally unrelated to the transplant may stir up unpleasant memories, leaving the patient shaken.

> "I used to get flashbacks for about a year after my transplant. I remember walking down the aisle of a grocery store, and I'd remember something about the transplant and get a big hit of adrenaline. But that pretty much ended when I made a conscious decision to stop worrying about relapse and the transplant."

During the first year after a transplant, some survivors find it hard to make long-term plans or commitments.

> "In the beginning, fear of relapse definitely affected my ability to make long-term commitments. I wouldn't start new projects or even pick out new clothes. I don't think I'll ever put it totally behind me, but I don't dwell on it anymore."

Many people who have been through the experience find it difficult to talk about, particularly with someone not intimately involved in the experience. They prefer to forget about the difficulties of the past, and go on with their lives.

Others want an outlet to talk about the experience. Support groups are helpful for some survivors, while others prefer one-on-one discussions with counselors, other transplant survivors, a family member or a friend. There are now chat rooms and discussion lists on the internet where patients and survivors can communicate with each other. You can contact BMT InfoNet at 888-597-7674 for the addresses of these sites or link to them through BMT InfoNet's web site at www.bmtinfonet.org/after/emotionalneeds.

> "The support group taught me how to talk about life's most difficult problems. The people in the group share the bond of an incredibly traumatic journey, and we're not afraid to help each other."

Family members and friends of transplant survivors may feel shut out by the patient who is unwilling to discuss her feelings with them. Although the patient may love them and appreciate their concern, patients need to cope with the transplant experience at their own pace and in their own way. Unfortunately, patients seldom have enough emotional energy to help both themselves and their loved ones deal with the experience, no matter how grateful they are for their support.

Despite the emotional upheaval a transplant causes, life after transplant can be very special. Survivors no longer take the future for granted, regardless of how promising their prognosis may be, and often enjoy each day of living more fully. As the months of survival turn into years, survivors experience the added pleasure of being able once again to look forward to many more years of life.

> "Each day is special for me. When I get up in the morning I look at the grass and trees and marvel at how beautiful everything is. For me, the transplant was like starting over again. It gave me a whole new life."

To learn more go to our web site at:

www.bmtinfonet.org/before/emotionalchallenges

Chapter Six

WHEN YOUR CHILD NEEDS A TRANSPLANT

It was like a whirlwind, a dream. One day our child was a normal 15-year-old boy who would live to be 80. The next day we were staring at blackboard diagrams about transplants, and hearing doctors tell us our son might die. It wasn't real. We didn't understand. All we could do was hug each other and cry.

Lorraine Boldt, mother of 11-year transplant survivor

"Your child needs a transplant" are some of the most difficult words a parent can hear. The uncertainty, feeling of helplessness, and emotional stress associated with deciding whether or not to proceed to transplant affects the entire family.

Young children may demonstrate rebellious or babyish behavior. Teens may express anger toward loved ones, engage in risky behavior or attempt to shut parents out. Young siblings may worry that they caused the child's disease or resent the extra attention he receives. Stress in marital relationships may intensify as everyone tries to cope with the difficult situation.

One thing is true: a transplant is a family affair. Acknowledging that everyone feels scared, but that everyone is working hard to make the child well can help the family pull together to face the challenges ahead. Sharing age-appropriate information with the child and siblings about the disease and treatment is important.

Through everything, remember this: thousands of children have been through a transplant and are now living normal, healthy lives.

Deciding on a Transplant

Choosing whether or not to proceed with a transplant is a difficult decision for families. The odds of success must be weighed against the certainty that the transplant will be a lengthy, rigorous procedure. There is often no clear-cut right choice, and parents and children can be frustrated about having to choose between several unpleasant options.

Getting easy-to-understand information prior to making a decision about a transplant is not always easy. Some transplant centers provide only oral explanations of what to expect, while others provide written materials, such as this book. The amount of information you receive can be overwhelming. It helps to have more than one adult present during meetings with medical personnel and to keep a journal of notes.

Sometimes parents receive conflicting information from their referring physician and the transplant team. The doctors may quote different survival rates or disagree about the timing of the transplant. Often, parents are not told about all the complications associated with a transplant until they meet with the transplant team.

> "The first conference with the transplant team was the most depressing experience of my life — worse than when my daughter was diagnosed. The doctor that referred us to the transplant center never told us about the possible side effects. I was terrified. I just wanted to grab my child and run."

Don't be shy about asking questions, even if you feel it's the hundredth time the question has been asked. Bring a written list of questions to your meeting with doctors and keep asking until you feel you have enough information to make a decision. It is the medical team's job to make sure all questions are answered, no matter how long or how many repetitions it takes.

Many parents find it helpful to talk to other parents whose child went through a transplant. BMT InfoNet's Caring Connections program can put you in contact with other parents. You can phone 888-597-7674 or access this service online at www.bmtinfonet.org/services/support. Keep in mind, however, that despite their similarities, no two families' experiences will be exactly alike.

Let your child ask questions as well. It is important to involve the child in the decision making process and secure his cooperation and trust.

Parents, particularly if their child is under age 14, are responsible for making the final decision in most states. Nonetheless, they know it is the child who must live with the consequences and this can create internal turmoil.

> "I knew it was a do or die situation but I kept asking myself, 'Do I really have the right to decide his life? I want to keep him with me as long as possible. Am I deciding what's best for me or for him?' "

Disagreements between parents, or between parents and children, about the wisdom of proceeding with a transplant are common.

> "We had just gotten our son back to the point where he seemed happy and healthy and now they were proposing a transplant. I kept thinking, 'Why take him back to ground zero? Why can't we leave him alone?' "

"Listen to each other carefully," advises a transplant nurse who has witnessed many such disagreements. "Respect others' concerns as much as your own."

It's a Family Affair

Once a decision has been made to proceed with a transplant, the treatment should be carefully explained to siblings. Involving siblings in discussions about your child's disease and treatment early on helps unite the family. It may also make siblings feel less resentful about the attention the sick child receives.

> "We decided our 12-year-old son and his brother would be told honestly about what was happening, and both would participate in decision-making as much as their age and maturity allowed. Although this placed a burden of maturity on both sons, they rose to meet it and our family drew closer, frequently drawing support from each other."

Families who involve siblings in discussions about the child's care and treatment often have fewer problems later on with sibling jealousy or anger. Be completely honest with both the child and siblings from the start so there are no surprises down the road and no feelings that they've been lied to, say psychologists who work with transplant patients.

Siblings often feel neglected or not loved as much as the child undergoing the transplant. SuperSibs! (Supersibs.org) offers programs to support siblings of cancer patients.

Questions Children Ask

Children's questions and concerns about the transplant vary depending on their age. Younger children focus on immediate problems like how much it will hurt, whether they will be separated from their parents, and when they can return to school. They may ask when their hair will grow back and whether or not they'll vomit a lot.

If they've received prior treatment for their disease, they may worry about whether they will have to have chemotherapy again. After acquiring a basic understanding of the procedure, younger children tend to rely on their parents to decide what's best.

Teens, on the other hand, take a much more active role in the decision-

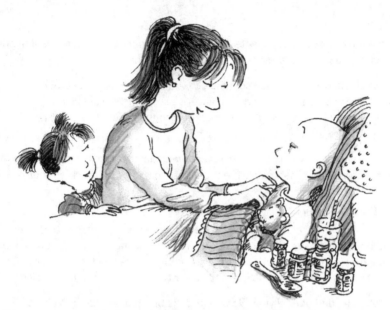

making process and, by law, must give their consent to the procedure in most states. They tend to be very concerned about self-image, and focus on issues like losing their hair. They worry about fitting back in with their peers once the transplant is over.

The possibility of infertility after transplant can be distressing for an adolescent. Sexual identity and activity are important to teens. Many don't understand the distinction between being fertile and being sexually active.

"Teens need help distinguishing between fertility and sexuality," says one psychologist. "It helps to tell them that many adults are infertile, yet lead a normal sex life. It's also important to help them distinguish between childbearing and child rearing."

Before undergoing a transplant, children should be introduced to the hospital, the transplant team, and the equipment that will be used during the procedure. It helps to show children unfamiliar devices like the catheters and IV poles. They should be given simple, clear explanations about what these devices do, why they are needed, and what it will feel like when they are used. Allowing younger children to handle the hospital equipment and try out the procedures on dolls before they enter the hospital often helps them get comfortable with the equipment, and allows them to ask questions.

Bringing siblings to the hospital and showing them where their brother or sister will spend the next several weeks is also a good idea. They will feel less left out, and will have a better sense of where their sibling will be and what will be done.

Coping With Anxiety

Once preparations for the transplant have been finalized, families can feel uneasy. Everyone will be anxious, and parents may agonize over the wisdom of proceeding with this treatment.

> "You have to learn to have confidence in your ability to make decisions, and believe you made the best choice under the circumstance. Don't panic about what may happen, and don't fret about what has happened. It can't be changed. Just take one day at a time."

For most children, the transplant will be the hardest challenge they've ever faced. Younger children may fear that they themselves are to blame for the disease and treatment. They may think they were somehow bad and are now being punished. Young siblings may also fear that they caused the problem. They may recall getting angry with the sick child and wishing the child would die, and now it is coming to pass.

It's important that children of all ages be encouraged to discuss their feelings openly so their concerns can be addressed. Find out what your child is thinking. Don't assume that if he doesn't talk about the illness or transplant, there's no problem. Some children express their anxieties by behavioral changes such as belligerence, depression, or poor performance in school. Let them know that you understand they're unhappy, frightened and confused, and that you are unhappy, too. Assure them that everyone will work hard to make them well again.

Sometimes children will more openly discuss their feelings with someone other than their parents. This is particularly true of adolescents who are fearful of hurting their parents' feelings or causing them distress. Adolescents who are coping with typical teen desires for independence may be especially reluctant to let down their guard in the presence of parents. While you may resent this, it's important to allow your child to discuss her feelings with whomever she feels most comfortable. You can seek the help of nurses, psychologists or other counselors to encourage your child to talk about her concerns.

Life During Transplant

Although a transplant is anything but routine, it is important to maintain as much of your child's normal home routine as possible. Bringing favorite clothes, pictures, and toys to the hospital helps maintain a sense of normalcy. Arranging for calls, letters and/or visits from your child's classmates, favorite teacher, church members, or a hometown doctor with whom your child feels comfortable can also help. Some families make videos of family and friends that the child can view while in the hospital.

Boredom in the hospital can be a big issue for children. Bringing favorite toys

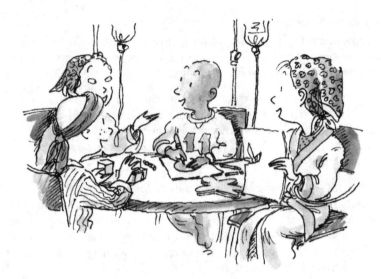

and games from home helps to ease the boredom. Planning diversions and activities for teens is especially important.

> "My son, who was 15 years old, was transplanted at a children's hospital. Although they had lots of activities planned, they were usually geared toward younger kids, not teens."

Loss of Control

Despite everyone's best efforts, the hospitalization will be a very stressful time for child and parents alike. The child will be inundated with tests, medications and daily medical procedures.

Children of all ages, and teens in particular, feel overwhelmed by all the rules and bosses, and can become angry over the loss of personal control. This can manifest itself in a variety of ways. Some become angry or belligerent, refusing to cooperate with parents or the medical staff. Others will cry for no apparent reason and may be unable to explain what is making them sad.

Some children refuse to eat or play. Still others may become depressed, listless or exhibit regressive or babyish behavior. They may be incapable of performing tasks they were previously able to do on their own. Parents usually bear the brunt of the behavioral changes.

"Children spend a whole lot of time and energy growing up, seizing control over their lives, and becoming more independent," explains one psychologist. "When they undergo a transplant, they lose that independence and control, and that can make them angry or depressed."

"Children don't feel the same urgency about routine medical procedures as parents do," notes a transplant nurse. "It's important to talk with children and let them know that you know it's hard, and to let them know that feeling angry is normal and okay."

> "I never said to my son, 'don't cry'. I encouraged him to talk about what was bothering him and to let it all out. If he really rebelled against doing something like mouth care, I wouldn't insist it be done that moment. We'd talk about it and usually it would get done without a fight five minutes later. Sometimes I'd suggest we do it a few minutes before the nurse came in so that he could feel like it was his decision and not her order that made it happen. He liked that feeling of control."

Children are as concerned about protecting their bodies and having control over their personal lives as adults, says one child therapist.

"Don't violate their bodies without asking permission. Give them the opportunity to say no or to make choices regarding their care or daily activities whenever it's possible for you to honor their decision."

Setting up and sticking to a daily routine in the hospital is important for children. Ideally, the routine should include some safe time for the child each day during which no unpleasant tests, medications, or staff interventions occur. One child's parents created a safe area for the child in the hospital room by bringing in a free-standing tent. When the child needed time alone, she would go into the tent to play.

Preparing for Medical Procedures

Preparing children for each new medication or medical procedure is very important. Children need to know what will be done, what the equipment will look like, and how they will feel during the procedure. Children should be told about the medication or procedure far enough in advance to allow them to work through questions, but not so far in advance that they have time to brood about it.

It helps to allow children to rehearse medical procedures in advance, or to practice the procedure on dolls or adults. Break the procedure into small steps, moving on to the next step only after the child's anxiety about the first step has been relieved.

Advance explanation is even required before the administration of drugs designed to ease pain or sedate the child.

> "The first time my child was given Demerol® he became almost violent. He wasn't prepared for the fact that he'd feel groggy and it frightened him. After that, I always made sure he knew in advance how the drugs would make him feel."

Parents can be important advocates for their children, particularly when it comes to securing pain relief or minimizing the discomfort associated with medical procedures. Some centers, for example, usually administer sedatives or other pain control medications to children in advance of a bone marrow aspirate while others do not. Don't hesitate to ask for pain medication if your child has difficulty with a procedure, and don't feel intimidated if the medical staff resists your request without providing a good reason.

Challenges for Parents

The time in the hospital is difficult for parents as well. It's hard to watch your child undergo difficult medical procedures, particularly when you have so little control over her care.

> "They kept saying that being there for my child was important but it never felt like I was doing enough."

It is important for you to pace yourself during this time so that you don't become exhausted or ill. Taking a few minutes or hours off while social workers or visitors spend time with your child can be helpful. Some parents find that spending the night away from the hospital enables them to get a good night's rest and better cope with the next day's stresses. For other parents, remaining with the child overnight is less stressful.

> "My mother and sister would sometimes stay with my son while I went to a nearby mall or got my hair done. Just getting outside, even for a few minutes, made a tremendous difference."

> "At first it was hard for me to leave my child each night, and I tried to get the hospital to change their policy. But it became a haven for me — I could take a hot bath, watch television, sleep and have some time to myself."

Children are very perceptive about their parents' feelings and can be frightened when they detect sadness or stress in their parents. Some children may feel guilty, thinking they caused their parents' sadness, and a desire to protect their parents can be a stumbling block to speaking frankly about their own concerns. Acknowledging that the hospitalization is scary for everyone involved and that you will work through the experience together is important.

> "Every day my son would say, 'I love you. Thank you for being here with me. It makes it easier when I'm not feeling good.' He knew it was just as hard for me as it was for him."

Siblings' Care

Often siblings must be left in the care of friends or relatives while their brother or sister is undergoing a transplant. This may involve removing them from their home and normal routines, especially if the transplant will take place out of town. Young children may view this separation from their parents as a punishment. It is important that siblings know that their parents don't want to be away from them, that the separation will be temporary, and why it's not possible for the siblings to be with their parents.

Setting up a plan of routine contact between the parents and siblings will help them feel they are not being ignored, or that they aren't loved as much as the sick child.

> "Every day I would call my daughter and write her a note. When I wrote, I would tell her what was happening with her brother, but when I called, I made sure we talked about her."

Marital Stress

It is not unusual for problems that previously existed in a home or marriage to be heightened during this time. Plans for a separation or divorce may get put on hold as a result of the transplant, with tensions between marital partners increasing. Substance abuse problems may become worse as a result of the added stress.

Don't be embarrassed to seek help for these problems — you won't be the first. In general, it's best to make as few changes as possible in the home routine and keep lines of communication open during this difficult time.

Even parents who previously felt they had a good relationship can experience severe marital tensions. Often, one parent — usually the mother — remains at the hospital with the child, while the spouse spends most of his time at home, continuing to work, taking care of the home and caring for the other children. Both may be thrust into roles they normally don't assume.

The caregiver at the hospital must deal with complicated medical issues, a child who is physically and emotionally exhausted, and her own exhaustion and emotions. She gets little or no break from the stress.

The spouse at home may assume more child care and household responsibilities, and must deal with his own fears as well as the emotional needs of his other children. He may feel left out or poorly informed about the day-to-day medical aspects of what's happening with the sick child.

Both parents are under stress and need each other's support. However, both are often too exhausted or upset to understand how their spouse feels and what he or she needs. As one mother put it, "Stress like this will either make a marriage stronger or pull it apart."

> "I was at the hospital 24 hours a day. My husband was able to re-enter the world when he became overwhelmed, go to the office, pretend to live a normal life. When we came home, he wanted things to return to normal, but I was just starting to look back and

process what we had been through. I was coping with the anger and fear I couldn't focus on in the hospital. I was extremely angry that he couldn't see things the way I did. One night I felt like our marriage was over. I told him he didn't understand where I'd been. He said, 'I've been there, too.' We went to therapy together and were able to address a lot of issues."

"I was a raving lunatic and my husband didn't understand why. I was dead tired and would have liked for him to pick up the slack. He couldn't do it. He was devastated when our child got sick — he'd never had to handle a catastrophe like this before. Sometimes, I just needed a big hug from him but he wasn't capable of it. I got mad and snippy with him when he wouldn't do little things like taking out the garbage without being asked. I started to resent him. I finally realized that if you have bad feelings, you have to talk about it even if your husband isn't a talker. It takes work to keep a marriage together under these circumstances. It's not a piece of cake."

"It's important to respect each other's differences. I think men and women handle crises in different ways. My husband and I handled our fears differently. One way is not necessarily better than the other."

Going Home

Going home — the day that everyone waits for — can be a bittersweet experience. Although the hospitalization has ended, the recovery period is far from over. Medications must be administered several times daily, catheters must be cleaned, and several visits per week must be made to the outpatient clinic to monitor progress. Parents will be on pins and needles watching for signs of infection or other complications.

"You think you'll get to go home and lead a normal life but it's not like that. Living at home with a child who has a weak immune system is scary. We were constantly worrying that my husband would bring home germs from work, and we carried disinfectant everywhere."

It is common for problems to develop that require the child to be re-admitted to the hospital for a short time. This can be alarming for parents and children alike.

"You never know what will come up. Since we've come home, we've had many trips to the hospital. There's still a lot of home care for our daughter, even now. She still has the central line, the feeding tube, and lots of medications to take. Every time something goes wrong I feel guilty, thinking that something I did made my child worse. Wrong thoughts, I know, but we're only human."

Sometimes, behavioral problems surface after transplant. "Parents are set up to be in an awkward position," explains one nurse. "While in the hospital, the child usually gets lots of cards, gifts, balloons and attention, and may expect it to continue when he returns home."

Frequently, friends and extended family fail to understand that the trauma continues long after a child returns home.

> "They think that once you walk out the door of the hospital,
> everything is behind you, and you should pick up life where
> you left off. It just doesn't work that way."

> "It would really drive me crazy when people would say, 'You must
> feel so lucky,' or 'You must be so grateful,' when I was feeling any-
> thing but lucky. While I was grateful to have witnessed a miracle,
> I was still really angry that our family had to go through all this."

The reunion of the siblings with the parent who spent time at the hospital with the transplant child is not always a smooth one.

> "At first my three-year-old refused to talk to me. My daughter was
> left in my husband's care at home during my son's transplant. She
> talked with my husband and treated him like her parent, but closed
> up to me. That hurt a lot. We found a therapist who helped us un-
> derstand her fears and resentments, and work through them."

Siblings can become jealous about the extra attention the transplant survivor receives after returning home. They may express a desire to be sick so their mother will pay more attention to them. They can resent the fact that differ-ent rules apply to them than to the transplant child.

Some parents have found that involving siblings in the routine caregiving can make them feel needed and important. Setting aside time for the parent and sibling to do something special together also helps.

> "My four-year-old daughter was not pleased when my son came
> home from the hospital. There was a lot of whining, crying and
> naughtiness like biting. She directed her anger at me, not my son.
> I tried to find special things for her — like special times for her to
> be with her parents or special treats when we'd take my son to
> the clinic. That seemed to help."

> "My five-year-old cried a lot. She kept asking, 'Why is my sister
> always sick? Why does she get extra attention?' I told her that
> I loved them equally, and I talked with her about what it was like
> when she was a little baby like her sister. I told her mommy was
> with her the whole time and paid lots of attention to her. I said, 'It's

okay to be angry, but it's not your sister's fault — don't be angry with her.' I feel like I missed a good bit of my five-year-old because I was so preoccupied with the baby and her problems from birth. Now I try to make up the difference in healthy ways."

The child undergoing a transplant often senses the sadness siblings feel over the lack of attention shown them. Said one little boy to his sister, "I'm sorry I'm so lazy right now and mom's doing everything for me. As soon as I feel better you can have mommy for awhile."

Getting Back to Normal

Getting back to normal will be a slow process. For many months after the transplant, both the transplant survivor and siblings may become anxious over symptoms of a common cold or other minor discomforts.

"I went to my son's room one night when I heard him sniffling. 'This feels so familiar,' he said. 'I always used to get sick at night and you'd have to take me to the hospital.' When I assured him that he would be okay, he said, 'That sounds familiar, too.' "

"Our daughter was afraid to get sick after her brother's transplant. When she got the flu last week it was the first time that she was the sick one rather than her brother. He hovered over her, rubbed her back, and brought her something to drink, trying to soothe her. They were both very concerned."

"Don't ignore or trivialize a sibling's complaints of illness," advises a transplant nurse. "Show them you are as concerned about their well-being as you are about the child who has had a transplant. Call the doctor even if you think it is something minor. It can help put their mind at ease."

"Don't assume siblings' complaints of illness are a deliberate ploy to get attention," advises a psychologist. "Children often mimic symptoms of the illness unconsciously, and truly believe they are ill."

Certain events that parents view as milestones can be very traumatic for the child. A two-year-old, for example, became very upset when his central line was removed. "We thought he'd be happy to get rid of it. Instead, he became very upset — it was like part of his body was being removed," said one mother.

Returning to school is a milestone that children are often encouraged to look forward to, but it, too, can be a tremendous letdown. They may find their classmates are not anxiously awaiting their return. Their friends have moved on to new interests and activities without them. Some children may be afraid to associate with a child who has been sick and now looks different.

It helps to prepare classmates in advance for the child's return. A nurse, doctor or social worker can visit the school, explain what has happened to the child, and answer questions. Even with advance preparation, however, the child who survives a transplant sometimes finds it difficult to fit back in. The Leukemia and Lymphoma Society offers a package of materials to help parents and teachers prepare children for the return of a classmate who has been ill.

Despite the difficulties, the transplant experience often brings families closer together:

> "My children still squabble a lot, but they're very concerned and protective of each other as well. It was rough while we went through it, but the good times have come now. My son made it, he's healthy, and we all appreciate what it means to be alive."

To learn more go to our web site at:

www.bmtinfonet.org/before/pediatrictransplants

Chapter Seven
PREPARATIVE REGIMEN

The doctor spent thirty minutes telling me all the things that could go wrong. Suddenly I could hear no more. 'Stop,' I said emphatically. 'I know you have to give me all the statistics, but I am not a statistic. My name is Harvey Erlich and I have an attitude problem. I refuse to die. Now, I believe that I can make it, do you?'

Harvey Erlich, three-year transplant survivor

The preparative regimen (also called the conditioning regimen) is the high-dose chemotherapy and/or radiation administered to patients during the week before their transplant.

The preparative regimen is designed to destroy as many diseased cells as possible without major damage to the patient's organs and tissues. Drugs used in the preparative regimen are sometimes the same as those used in standard chemotherapy to treat the disease. The dosages, however, are much higher and therefore more effective in killing the disease.

The high-dose chemotherapy and radiation also destroy the stem cells in the bone marrow. Therefore, an infusion of stem cells is required to rescue the patient from the effects of the preparative regimen, even if the disease being treated has not spread to the bone marrow.

High-Dose Chemotherapy

Most preparative regimens include high-dose combination chemotherapy. The chemotherapy drugs are usually administered intravenously over a two to four day period through a catheter that has been previously installed in a large vein near the chest. If the chemotherapy drug busulfan is part of your preparative regimen, it may be administered intravenously or taken as a pill.

Total Body Irradiation (TBI)

Some preparative regimens include total body irradiation. TBI is used most often in transplants for patients with leukemia, lymphoma and multiple myeloma. Total body irradiation is typically administered to patients in one or more sessions over a one to seven day period. When TBI is administered over several days it is called fractionated TBI. More than one session of TBI each day is called hyperfractionated TBI.

While patients do not actually see or feel the radiation, many still find TBI therapy an unnerving experience. Patients must sit or lie still, sometimes in an awkward position, for 10 to 45 minutes while the radiation is being administered. This can be difficult, particularly if the patient is nauseated. Some transplant centers use special stands or boxes to help patients remain immobile during TBI. These can be confining and make some patients feel anxious.

Pre-medication with sedatives can help reduce anxiety. Children are usually sedated before TBI sessions in an effort to minimize their movement and very young children may even be given anesthesia.

It helps to visit the radiation center before TBI therapy begins in order to familiarize yourself with the equipment and to get your questions answered. Some centers provide patients with a simulation of TBI therapy so they know in advance what to expect, and so that the health care team can assure that dosages and equipment measurements are correct.

Side Effects

High-dose chemotherapy and TBI are toxic to normal tissues and organs, as well as diseased cells. Nausea, vomiting, diarrhea, mouth sores and temporary hair loss almost always occur to varying degrees regardless of which preparative regimen is used. Severe or long-term damage to organs and tissues occurs less frequently.

Patients are often frightened and overwhelmed by the list of possible side effects associated with the preparative regimen. Keep in mind that most side effects are temporary and completely reversible, and that severe or long-term problems are the exception rather than the rule. Moreover, most discomfort associated with side effects can usually be prevented or relieved with medication.

As you read the following sections, keep in mind that the degree to which people experience side effects is different, and no one experiences all possible side effects.

Nausea, Vomiting and Diarrhea

Nausea and vomiting are common following all preparative regimens, but can be controlled with medications. Drugs called antiemetics are used to treat nausea. (Emesis means vomiting; thus, antiemetics are drugs that prevent vomiting.)

Antiemetics can cause side effects such as anxiety, drowsiness and restlessness. Occasionally, muscle tightness, uncontrolled eye movement or shakiness can occur. These drug reactions can be frightening, but are usually less serious than they appear. Lowering the dosage of the antiemetic, or administering an antihistamine usually reduces or eliminates the problem.

Diarrhea following the preparative regimen is also common. Anti-diarrheal drugs such as Lomotil® sedate the nerves in the gastrointestinal area, slowing down muscle contractions and the diarrhea.

Mouth, Throat, Skin and Hair

High-dose chemotherapy and radiation target rapidly dividing cells, such as cancer cells. However, some normal cells also divide rapidly such as those that line the mouth, throat and gut, as well as hair and skin cells. These cells can be temporarily damaged by high-dose chemotherapy or radiation.

Mouth sores (mucositis) and throat sores (stomatitis) typically appear four to eight days following the preparative regimen. Topical anesthetics such as Dyclone®, or narcotics such as morphine, are used to relieve this discomfort. Frequent brushing of teeth and gums with a soft brush or sponge, and rinsing with a solution of saline helps prevent mouth infections.

Mucositis often makes eating difficult or impossible. Patients may be fed intravenously until the discomfort subsides. Intravenous feeding is also used if the stomach is unable to absorb sufficient nutrients as a result of temporary irritation caused by the preparative regimen. Antacid medication may be given to counteract stomach irritation. (For more on eating difficulties after transplant, see Chapter Ten, Nutrition.)

Temporary hair loss (alopecia) occurs following the preparative regimen. Hair loss changes a patient's appearance and for some can be very distressing. Scarves, hats or wigs can be used until the hair grows back. Some patients prefer to shave their heads or cut their hair very short before hair loss begins. Hair normally grows back within three to six months following the transplant. Sometimes the amount of curl or thickness of the new hair will differ from the patient's hair pre-transplant. In rare cases, hair loss may be permanent.

Skin rash is common following preparative regimens that include TBI, busulfan, etoposide, carmustine or thiotepa. At some centers showers are recommended one and six hours after infusion of thiotepa to reduce the likelihood of developing a rash.

Less often, hyperpigmentation – dark spots on the skin – occur. They usually fade over a period of one to two months.

Bladder Irritation (hemorrhagic cystitis)

Bladder irritation, sometimes evidenced by bloody or painful urination, can occur following the preparative regimen, particularly those that include cyclo-phosphamide or ifosfamide. Increasing the rate of intravenous fluids, using a catheter to irrigate the bladder, and/or administering a drug called MESNA® are techniques commonly used to prevent or treat this problem.

Liver, Lungs and Heart

Temporary organ damage can occur following high-dose chemotherapy TBI. It is usually both mild and completely reversible.

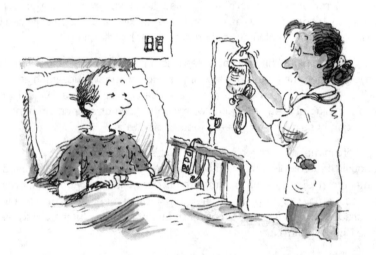

Liver blood test abnormalities occur in approximately 50 percent of patients following the preparative regimen, but only a small fraction actually develop liver damage. Patients may experience jaundice (yellowing of the skin), signifi-cant weight gain due to fluid retention, and abnormal blood levels of liver en-zymes and bilirubin (a pigment produced during the break up of red blood cells). Resting the liver and avoiding medications that aggravate the condition are the usual treatments until the liver heals itself. (For more on liver prob-lems following transplant, see Chapter Nine, Liver Complications.)

Breathing irregularities can also occur following the preparative regimen. Some patients develop pneumonia during the first four weeks after transplant. In most cases, injury to the lungs is mild and temporary, but some patients do experience long-term breathing problems.

Mild, temporary heartbeat irregularities (arrhythmia) or rapid heartbeat can occur following the preparative regimen, particularly those that include cyclophosphamide or carmustine. Severe or long-term heart problems are very rare.

Confusion

Confusion or altered thinking is an occasional, temporary side effect of the preparative regimen, or of drugs used to control other side effects. Confusion and altered thinking can be frightening both to the patient and their loved ones who observe it. It helps to remember that these problems are temporary and reversible, and can usually be managed by changing the dosage or type of drug.

Muscle Spasms and Cramping

Muscle spasms are a common problem after transplant. They may be caused by an imbalance in electrolytes — minerals found in the body such as potassium, magnesium and calcium. These minerals must be maintained at certain levels to prevent organ malfunction.

Muscle spasms can often be resolved by taking potassium, calcium, magnesium or phosphate supplements. Ask your doctor to prescribe the supplement, since not all sources of these minerals are absorbed equally well by the body. If there is no electrolyte imbalance, vitamin E or quinine in pill form sometimes resolves or reduces the problem.

Reproductive Organs

Damage to reproductive organs from high-dose chemotherapy or radiation is common, and usually results in permanent infertility. Patient age, gender, stage of sexual maturity, and the dosage of TBI or chemotherapy, all affect the likelihood of becoming infertile after transplant. In addition, women often experience premature menopause. (For more about infertility after transplant, see Chapter Thirteen, Sexuality after Transplant and Chapter Fourteen, Family Planning.)

Other Long-Term Side Effects

Premature cataracts occur in approximately 20 percent of patients who undergo fractionated TBI. Cataracts may also occur following treatment with high-dose busulfan. Cataracts can be surgically removed, usually in an outpatient setting.

Some patients experience numbness and tingling in their hands and feet, due to nerve damage caused by the preparative regimen or prior chemotherapy. Usually the damage is permanent. However, in a few patients there has been slow re-growth of nerve tissue that eventually reduces the problem.

Mild to moderate learning disabilities and memory problems may occur, especially if the preparative regimen included TBI.

Young children often experience delayed growth as well. Hormone therapy may promote growth. After chemotherapy, children should be followed by a pediatrician with specific knowledge of growth problems.

Children transplanted before the age of five may also experience significant dental problems, such as loose teeth, tooth loss, dry mouth and may be unable to wear braces. It is important that they be followed by a dentist who is experienced in treating children who've undergone high-dose chemotherapy or TBI. Similar problems can occur in adults who receive TBI. Routine dental check ups are recommended to prevent or correct these problems.

Putting Risks Into Perspective

Anxiety about the possible side effects is normal. It helps to put the risk of developing each side effect into perspective, and to remember that most are temporary and completely reversible. Counselors and psychiatrists are available at most transplant centers to help patients cope with their anxiety. It pays to take advantage of these resources.

> "Be prepared for complications. Very few things will happen just as described. There are many possible complications. No one gets all of them, but most get some of them. Learn to separate those that are serious, but reversible, from those that are truly life-threatening."

To learn more go to our web site at:

www.bmtinfonet.org/during/prepregimen

Chapter Eight
INFECTION

Six months after my transplant, I developed a herpes zoster infection, also known as shingles. I was hospitalized for ten days. That was hard. I was just getting back on my feet and wham! — I'm back in the hospital again.

Marilyn Rossen, 11-year transplant survivor

The air we breathe, the food we eat, the items we touch — everything we contact in daily life is a potential source of bacteria, viruses or fungi that can cause infection. For a normal, healthy individual these daily encounters with sources of infection are not a major problem. Our immune system protects us.

For transplant patients, however, it's a different story. The high-dose chemotherapy or radiation administered prior to transplant cannot distinguish between diseased and normal cells. Not only are diseased cells destroyed, but the patient's immune system is disrupted as well.

Skin and mucous membranes (lining of the mouth, nose and intestines), which are the body's first line of defense against infection, may be damaged. White blood cells, part of the body's internal defense team, are destroyed. (This condition is called neutropenia.)

Special proteins called antibodies that normally help destroy bacteria and viruses are depleted. Until the transplanted stem cells engraft and produce new white blood cells, patients are extremely vulnerable to infection.

The first two to four weeks after a transplant are a particularly critical time. Although the risk of infection steadily declines once the stem cells begin producing new white blood cells, the patient's immune system usually remains compromised — not functioning at 100 percent efficiency — for six months to a year after the transplant.

Although post-transplant infections are a serious cause for concern, great strides have been made to better manage and prevent them.

Bacterial Infections

Bacteria are microscopic organisms that invade tissues and multiply rapidly. Bacteria can cause infections anywhere in the body and are the usual cause of ear and sinus infections, as well as bronchitis.

Bacteria secrete poisonous chemicals called toxins that interfere with normal organ functions. Toxins can, among other things, cause shock or low blood pressure that can lead to death if sufficient oxygen is not provided to the heart or brain.

Bacteria can also disrupt normal organ functions by their sheer number. Some pneumonias, for example, are caused by rapidly multiplying bacteria that fill up the spaces in lungs where air is normally absorbed into the body.

Bacterial infections are most common during the first two to four weeks after transplant and occur in 20 percent of patients. The infections occur most often in the intestines, on the skin and in the mouth. They also occasionally occur in the bladder or lungs.

To combat bacterial infections, large doses of antibiotics are usually given during the first few weeks after transplant if the patient's temperature rises above 100.5°F. Patients bathe or shower daily to remove bacteria from their skin. Soft toothbrushes or sponges are used to cleanse the gums and teeth so that cuts, through which infectious agents may enter, can be avoided.

Hospital staff and others who come in contact with patients carefully wash their hands with antiseptic soap prior to touching the patient, since hands are a primary carrier of infection. Flowers and plants (both live and dried) which can harbor harmful bacteria or fungi are usually not permitted in the room while the patient's immune system is weak. Similarly, fresh fruits and vegetables may be eliminated from the patient's diet until his immune system is functioning normally. When detected promptly and treated with antibiotics, bacterial infections are seldom fatal.

Fungal Infections

Fungi are primitive life forms that we encounter daily. Mold on bread is an example of a common fungus. Most are harmless and some, such as the fungus called Candida, normally reside inside our bodies.

Fungal infections are less common than bacterial infections in the first few weeks after transplant, but are very difficult to treat. Unfortunately, while the widespread use of antibiotics after transplant has successfully reduced the incidence of harmful bacterial infections, these antibiotics can also destroy beneficial bacteria in the body that keep fungi in check.

At some transplant centers, special air-filtering equipment is installed in patient hospital rooms to remove fungi from the air. Eliminating fresh plants, fruits and vegetables from the patient's environment also may also reduce the risk of fungal infections.

Candida and aspergillus are the most common fungal infections after transplant. Candida live in the intestines, mouth and vagina and are normally kept in check by bacteria. When bacteria are destroyed by antibiotics, however, the fungi can multiply and spread, infecting many parts of the body.

Aspergillus infections occur most often in sinus passages or the lungs, and can cause pneumonia. The aspergillus fungus is frequently found around construction sites or where buildings are being remodeled.

Patients who have continuous fevers after taking antibiotics are usually given an anti-fungal drug called amphotericin B. A drug called fluconazole is often used to prevent Candida infections.

Aspergillus infections are difficult to treat and can be life threatening. New techniques used to diagnose aspergillus infections earlier, as well as the use of amphotericin B and fluconazole, have helped reduce the number of deaths from aspergillus infections.

Once blood counts return to normal levels, the risk of fungal infection drops dramatically. Overall, serious fungal infections are rare following an autologous transplants.

Viral Infections

Viruses are tiny parasites, smaller than bacteria, that are not self-sufficient. They must invade other organisms, such as human cells, in order to survive. Viruses tinker with the genetic machinery of the host cell, turning it into a factory for the production of more of the virus. The virus eventually destroys or cripples the host cell and moves on to neighboring cells to continue the process.

Infections caused by viruses are very difficult to treat. Several anti-viral agents such as acyclovir and ganciclovir are useful, but the number of viruses they effectively treat is small. Viral infections following transplant occur either as a result of exposure to a new virus or reactivation of an old virus that was already in the patient's body.

The risk of developing a serious viral infection following an autologous transplant is low. The viral infections that occur most are caused by the herpes simplex virus (HSV), varicella zoster virus (VZV), or cytomegalovirus (CMV).

Herpes Simplex

Herpes simplex infections are caused by two separate viruses: herpes I and herpes II. Although both can cause an infection in any part of the body, the herpes I virus usually causes painful fever blisters in and around the mouth. The herpes II virus usually causes painful blisters on the genitalia or rectum.

An estimated 70 percent of Americans are exposed to the herpes I virus, usually during childhood. The virus is highly contagious and is usually transmitted through contact with persons having active herpes sores on their mouths. Herpes II, on the other hand, is usually transmitted through sexual intercourse with an infected partner.

Herpes infections often recur after the initial episode. The virus can lay dormant in the body for many years, flaring up from time to time. Even if a person does not recall having had an active case of herpes, the virus may nonetheless be present in his body.

When a herpes infection occurs, it is usually during the first month after transplant. Herpes simplex responds well to treatment with anti-viral agents such as acyclovir. Most centers give patients acyclovir before a herpes infection develops which has greatly reduced the incidence of herpes infections after transplant.

Varicella Zoster Virus (VZV)

Varicella zoster virus (VZV) is often referred to as herpes zoster or shingles. It is the same virus that causes chicken pox. Twenty to 50 percent of patients develop a VZV infection during the first year after transplant, usually after the third month. VZV is seen most often in patients being treated for leukemia, lymphoma or Hodgkin disease.

VZV infections manifest themselves in one of two ways. An itching, blistering skin rash may develop and extend along any one of the body's nerve branches. The nerve endings under the skin at the site of the rash are infected and can cause great pain.

Alternatively, a VZV infection can develop in the nerve to the eye called the ophthalmic nerve. A painful rash may occur along the nerve path on the forehead and eyelids. If not treated promptly, the infection can damage the eye.

VZV infections may be treated with oral doses of famciclovir or valcyclovir, or acyclovir given intravenously. They are quite contagious, and some patients must be admitted to the hospital to be treated.

The pain associated with a VZV infection can be significantly reduced if you call your doctor the day the rash first appears. Medications such as acetaminophen, codeine or morphine may be administered to control pain. Early treatment can significantly reduce the duration of VZV infections.

A VZV infection can occur more than once after transplant. The itching or pain associated with a VZV infection can continue long after all clinical signs of the disease disappear.

Since VZV infections are highly contagious, patients should avoid people with chicken pox or a VZV infection for the first year after transplant.

Cytomegalovirus (CMV)

CMV infections can develop in many organs, including the liver, colon, eyes or lungs. Although all CMV infections are cause for concern, CMV pneumonia is particularly worrisome because it is very difficult to treat. Most patients are given ganciclovir to prevent CMV infections.

Approximately one-third to one-half of the general population are exposed to CMV during their lifetime, particularly urban dwellers. Doctors can test a patient's blood to see if CMV is present prior to transplant. If it is not, the patient is CMV-negative, and care is taken to prevent exposure to CMV before, during and after the transplant. Filtering blood products given to patients to remove most of the white blood cells reduces the risk of developing a CMV infection.

Other Viruses

Other viruses such as adenovirus, papovavirus, Epstein-Barr virus (EBV), respiratory syncitial virus (RSV), and human papilloma virus (HPV) can also create problems after transplant, although the incidence of these infections is quite low.

Adenovirus and RSV infections can cause pneumonia. Adenovirus can cause an infection in the kidneys or gastrointestinal tract. Ribavirin is effective in treating both of these viruses.

The likelihood of developing viral infections can be greatly reduced by limiting contact with the public after transplant (particularly people with the flu or colds), and by meticulous hand washing. Some centers require a brief period of isolation from the general public after transplant to reduce the risk of viral infections.

Protozoa

Protozoa are single-cell parasites that feed on organisms such as human cells. Although protozoan infections are less common than bacterial or viral infections, they can pose serious problems for transplant patients.

One protozoan called pneumocystis carinii is found in the trachea (windpipe) of healthy human beings. When a person's immune system is suppressed, this protozoan may enter the lungs and grow into tiny cysts which cause pneumonia. Trimethoprim/sulfamethoxazole (Bactrim® or Septra®) and pentamidine are highly effective in preventing and treating pneumocystis carinii pneumonia.

Another infection called toxoplasmosis occasionally develops in patients after transplant. Toxoplasmosis is caused by a protozoan called toxoplasma gondii which is often in the feces of cats. Toxoplasmosis may infect the brain, eyes, muscles, liver and/or lungs. A painful, inflamed retina in the eye is a common manifestation of the disease which, without prompt treatment, can result in damage to the eye. With early diagnosis and treatment, toxoplasmosis is treatable.

Preventing Infection

Although it may be tempting to throw caution to the wind after a transplant, it's best not to take chances. Bacteria, viruses and fungi that are harmless to most people can cause a very serious infection in a patient whose immune system has not yet fully recovered.

Your medical team will give you guidelines to help you prevent infections. The most important of these is frequent hand washing with antibacterial soap and water or an alcohol-based hand sanitizer, especially in these circumstances:

- before eating or preparing food

- after changing diapers (if you are permitted to do so)

- after touching plants or dirt (if you are permitted to do so)

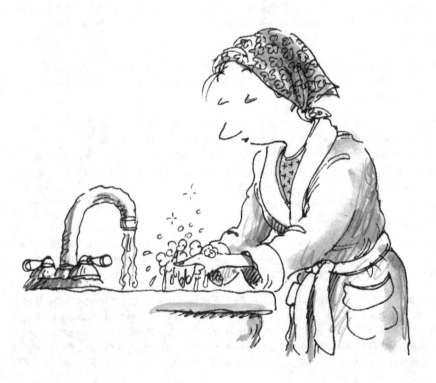

- after urinating or defecating

- after touching animals

- after touching bodily fluids or items that might have come in contact with bodily fluids such as clothing, bedding or toilets

- after going outdoors or to a public place

- after removing gloves

- after collecting or depositing garbage (if you are permitted to do so)

- before and after touching catheters and wounds

During the first six months after transplant, many transplant centers recommend that these additional precautions be observed:

- Avoid crowds or people who have infections

- Avoid people who have recently been vaccinated with chicken pox or polio

- Avoid changing a baby's diapers

- Avoid gardening

- Avoid walking, wading, swimming or playing in ponds or lakes

- Avoid construction sites and remodeling projects while you are at risk for infections

- Treat well water before drinking

If You Have Pets

Rules vary among transplant centers as to whether or not you can have pets in the home while you are recovering. Consult your transplant center for its guidelines which may include:

- Avoid contact with an animal that is ill

- Avoid adopting ill or juvenile pets (juvenile pets are more likely to scratch than mature pets)

- Avoid reptiles such as lizards, snakes, turtles and iguanas and items they touch

- Avoid chicks and ducklings

- Avoid exotic pets such as monkeys or chinchillas

- Feed pets only high quality commercial food or thoroughly cooked human food

- Avoid contact with animal feces; do not clean litter boxes or cages or dispose of animal waste

- Do not touch bird droppings. Use disposable gloves and a mask if you must be near bird droppings.

- Avoid cleaning fish tanks

- Do not place cat litter boxes in areas of the house where food is prepared or eaten

- Keep cats indoors and do not adopt stray cats

- Cover backyard sandboxes to prevent cats from using them as a litter box

At the first sign of fever or infection, call your physician. Infections are most easily treated when caught early. Infections you formerly ignored can be serious problems after transplant. Taking precautions to guard against infection can be a nuisance, but it can also save your life.

Re-vaccination

After an autologous transplant, it is possible that antibodies that previous protected you against disease may be depleted. The Centers for Disease Control suggest that patients be re-vaccinated for diphtheria, tetanus, pneumococcus, hemophilus, influenza, type B measles, mumps, rubella, and polio infections approximately a year-and-a-half after transplant. You should discuss this issue with your transplant doctor.

For more information go to our web site at:

www.bmtinfonet.org/after/preventinfections

Chapter Nine
LIVER COMPLICATIONS

I developed more complications than most people after my transplant, including kidney and liver problems. In August, they sent me home. Later, they told me I was the sickest patient they had ever discharged. Once I got home, though, I started to recuperate very quickly.

Jean Pfaendtner, 14-year transplant survivor

The liver is a complex organ that performs many essential functions. It removes toxins from the bloodstream, manufactures proteins that control blood clotting, stores energy, breaks down drugs, produces a fluid called bile that helps digestion, and rids the body of bilirubin — a pigment produced during the breakup of old red blood cells.

If the blood vessels that transport blood through the liver become blocked, or if the cells in the liver are damaged, the liver cannot properly rid the body of toxins, drugs, and other waste products. If the bile duct that connects the liver to the gallbladder becomes blocked, excess levels of bilirubin, cholesterol and other chemicals will build up in the body, interfering with organ function.

Liver disorders fall into three categories:

- those that affect the liver cells

- those that affect the vessels that transport blood through the liver

- those that affect the bile ducts that carry bile from the liver to the gallbladder and intestines

A patient who has undergone an autologous transplant may experience more than one liver disorder at the same time. While some are serious, the majority result in only mild or moderate liver damage that is temporary and reversible.

Patients who have had liver disorders prior to transplant are at greater risk of developing liver disorders after transplant. You will therefore be tested before transplant for evidence of fungal liver infections, hepatitis, and gallstones or other obstructions of the bile duct that may need to be removed before the transplant proceeds.

A variety of tests are used to determine whether liver disease is present. During treatment, the transplant staff will weigh you daily and may measure the your abdominal girth (like a waistline measurement, but around the abdomen instead). Blood tests will determine whether there is too much bilirubin or other liver enzymes in the blood. You will be examined daily for signs of jaundice or swelling that might indicate a liver problem.

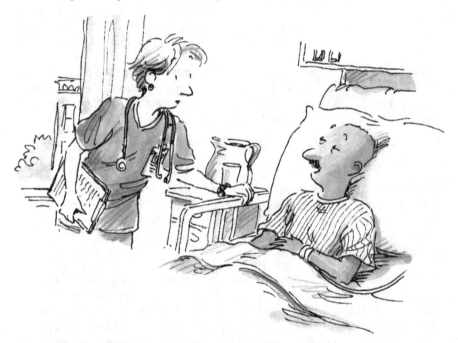

The First Three Months After Transplant

The liver complications described in the remainder of this chapter usually occur during the first three months following transplant unless otherwise noted.

Veno-Occlusive Disease (VOD)

Veno-occlusive disease is a potentially serious liver problem caused by high-dose chemotherapy or radiation. The blood vessels that carry blood through the liver become swollen and blocked. Without a supply of blood, the liver cannot remove toxins, drugs and other waste products from the bloodstream. Fluids build up in the liver causing swelling and tenderness. The kidneys may retain excess water and salt, causing swelling in the legs, arms and abdomen.

In severe cases of VOD, excess fluid in the abdominal cavity puts pressure on the lungs making it difficult to breathe. Toxins that are not processed out of the blood by the liver may affect how the brain functions and confusion may result (although confusion is a symptom of other, less serious problems as well).

Symptoms are usually first seen one to four weeks after the start of the preparative regimen. VOD can be difficult to diagnose, however, since its symptoms are signs of other liver disorders as well. If an enlarged liver *and* sudden weight gain *and* jaundice occur early after transplant and cannot be explained by other causes, the problem is probably VOD.

There currently is no proven therapy to prevent VOD. When a patient is diagnosed with VOD, the medical team may minimize or eliminate the use of certain drugs that aggravate the problem, remove excess fluid in tissues and organs with diuretics or dialysis, restrict salt intake, carefully monitor fluid volumes in the body, and transfuse the patient with red blood cells.

Patients with a history of hepatitis, as well as those who develop an infection and fever immediately before or during the course of the preparative regimen, have an increased risk of developing VOD. Patients undergoing a second transplant also may have an increased risk of developing VOD.

In most cases, VOD is mild or moderate, and the liver damage is reversible. Severe VOD, however, can be life threatening. Studies are underway to to find more effective ways to treat VOD.

Fungal Liver Disease

Fungal liver disease is a serious complication after transplant. If it occurs, it is usually during the first three months after transplant, although it can occur later, as well.

A candida infection, is the usual cause of fungal liver disease. In healthy individuals, the spread of Candida is kept in check by the immune system and by beneficial bacteria that reside in the body. However, antibiotics given to patients to destroy harmful bacteria also destroy the beneficial bacteria that keep the spread of Candida fungi in check.

Symptoms of fungal liver infection include persistent fever, a tender and swollen liver, and an elevated level of alkaline phosphatase in the blood. Patients with fungal infections in their intestine or bloodstream after transplant are at greatest risk of developing fungal liver disease. Patients who have persistent low neutrophil (also called granulocyte) counts are more likely to develop fungal liver infections than others.

Fungal infections are very difficult to treat, particularly when the immune system is weak. Amphotericin B and fluconazole are two drugs that have shown some effectiveness in treating fungal liver infection.

Liver Injury From Drugs

Several drugs administered to patients to treat infections, nausea, or high-blood pressure, as well as some sedatives and pain medications, can cause or aggravate liver injury. However, these drugs seldom cause severe liver damage. The signs of drug injury are jaundice and abnormal levels of bilirubin and liver enzymes in the blood.

Prolonged periods of intravenous feeding may also cause mild liver problems in transplant patients. These may include liver inflammation, abnormal bile flow and fat accumulation in the liver. Once the patient begins eating on his own, the liver problems resolve. If the patient is not able to eat on his own, varying the content of the intravenous feeding sometimes helps.

Viral Hepatitis

Occasionally, viral hepatitis (inflammation of the liver caused by a virus) occurs during the first three months after transplant. It is usually caused by the hepatitis C virus but can also be caused by other viruses such as adenovirus, herpes simplex virus, varicella zoster virus, echovirus, cytomegalovirus (CMV), and the Epstein-Barr virus.

Liver inflammation caused by the hepatitis B or C virus is usually mild. Transplant centers now screen blood products for CMV and the hepatitis A, B and C viruses, before infusing the blood into patients.

Liver infections caused by other viruses (adenovirus, herpes simplex virus, varicella zoster virus) rarely cause severe liver damage. Early diagnosis of these infections is important since therapies available to treat these viruses are most effective during the early stages of infection.

Chronic Viral Hepatitis

Viruses can linger in the body long after symptoms of acute infection disappear and infections can recur long after the first episode. This is particularly true if the body's immune system is not functioning normally as is the case with patients recovering from an autologous stem cell transplant.

Because viruses can be present in the body for many years without symptoms, some people who were transplanted or had blood transfusions before the early 1990s are now finding that they received transfusions containing the hepatitis C virus and are now infected. A small percentage of blood and platelet transfusions done in the 1970s and 1980s contained the virus, and no test was available until 1990 to detect it.

Tests are now available to determine if a person is infected with hepatitis C. The combination of interferon-alpha and ribavirin can, in some patients, eliminate hepatitis C virus from the bloodstream and improve the liver inflammation caused by the virus.

Biliary Disease

When patients stop eating for an extended period of time (e.g. when they are fed intravenously), the gallbladder, which stores bile and squeezes it into the intestine after meals, does not empty. The bile becomes thick and granular, creating biliary sludge. The sludge can obstruct the bile duct and interfere with the flow of bile to the small intestine.

Symptoms of this problem include pain after eating, inflammation of the gallbladder, fever, and gallstones. The problem usually resolves once the patient begins eating normally. In rare cases, an infection of the bile duct or inflammation of the pancreas may result.

Chapter Ten
NUTRITION

*After my transplant, I was the nausea queen. You name it, I could throw it up.
For awhile, all I could handle was Carnation Instant Breakfast®. Then I worked
my way up to Cap'n Crunch®— box after box of it — then coffee and beer, and
finally, at long last, a normal diet.*

Judith Miller, six-year transplant survivor

We all need food and water to thrive. The calories in food provide the fuel our
organs and tissues need to grow and function. Protein-rich foods enable the
body to build and repair muscle and body tissue. Vitamins and minerals keep
blood, skin and the nervous system functioning properly.

Transplant patients have unique nutritional requirements. Prior to transplant,
patients undergo high-dose chemotherapy and/or total body irradiation (TBI)
to destroy their disease. This severely stresses the body's organs and tissues.
In order to repair any organ or tissue damage that might occur and to fight
fever, patients need to increase their intake of calories and protein.

Typically, transplant patients require 50-60 percent more calories and twice
as much protein in their diets than healthy individuals of similar age and gender. The need for more calories and protein usually persists at least one to two
months after transplant.

Changing Diet Before Transplant

Some patients consider making major dietary changes before their transplant.
Some attempt to shed excess weight. Others increase their intake of foods
that have been associated with a lower incidence of cancer. Still others turn to
macrobiotic or other diets that restrict the types of foods consumed.

If you are considering changing your diet, ask your doctor for a referral to a registered dietitian who can evaluate the nutritional adequacy of the new diet. Some diets, such as macrobiotic diets, contain lower amounts of protein and other nutrients than are required by a recovering transplant patient.

Using certain herbs, roots or over the counter vitamins can be dangerous for people undergoing transplantation. Consult your doctor or dietitian before using these products.

Quick weight loss is also usually discouraged. Since patients often lose weight while undergoing treatment, limiting food intake before a transplant could cause a serious nutrient deficiency.

Several studies have suggested a relationship between types of foods consumed and the risk of developing cancer. However, no study has proven that changing your diet can cure cancer. Eating a balanced diet that is low in fat, contains lots of fresh fruits and vegetables and includes fiber from a variety of sources is a patient's best bet, say dieticians who work with transplant patients.

Nutrition After Transplant

For the first three months after transplant, patients are usually advised to avoid foods that may contain elements that could cause infection. Many transplant centers have specific recommendations on foods to avoid which may include:

- Raw or undercooked meat
- Dishes that contain undercooked meat such as sausages or casseroles
- Raw or undercooked eggs or foods that might contain them
- Raw or undercooked seafood, such as sushi
- Unroasted raw nuts or unshelled nuts
- Miso products
- Non-pasteurized milk products
- Cheeses with mold
- Soft cheeses such as brie or feta
- Smoked or pickled seafood
- Raw honey
- Tempe products

Consult your transplant team to learn which dietary restrictions apply to you.

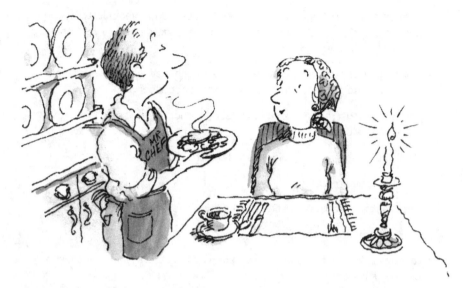

Consuming sufficient calories, protein and fluids can be difficult particularly during the first few weeks after transplant. Mouth sores, nausea, vomiting, dry mouth, diarrhea, constipation, depression and fatigue can make mealtimes unappealing. Certain medications can also cause a loss of appetite.

Some patients must be fed intravenously during this period to ensure they receive sufficient calories, protein, vitamins, minerals and fluids. The intravenous feeding is called total parenteral nutrition (TPN) or hyperalimentation and may supply all the patient's nutritional requirements or supplement those he is able to consume on his own.

Often, eating problems can be overcome without resorting to the use of TPN. The following sections describe common eating problems after transplant and suggestions for overcoming them.

Mouth and Throat Sores

Mouth and throat sores are common after transplant. They may be caused by chemotherapy, total body irradiation or infection. The sores can make eating painful, but the following suggestions may help:

- Eat foods lukewarm or cold, rather than hot.

- Cook foods until tender and soft.

- Drink through a straw to bypass mouth sores.

- Eat high-protein, high-calorie foods to speed healing of the sores.

- Try a liquid or blenderized diet, or a complete nutrition supplement such as Ensure®, Boost®, or Carnation Instant Breakfast®.

- Eat soft foods such as creamed soups, cheeses, mashed potatoes, yogurt, cooked eggs, custards, puddings, cooked cereals, ice cream, milk shakes and pasteurized eggnog.

- Eat cold foods such as milk shakes, cottage cheese, yogurt, watermelon, gelatin and soft, canned fruit (blenderized if necessary).

- Eat soft, non-irritating frozen foods such as popsicles, ice cream, frozen yogurt and slushes.

- Drink fruit nectars and fruit flavored beverages instead of acidic juices.

- Maintain good mouth care.

- Request pain medications if discomfort is severe.

If you develop mouth or throat sores, avoid:

- tart or acidic foods and beverages such as citrus fruits and juices, and pineapple juice

- salty foods (including broth)

- strong spices (such as peppers, chili powder, nutmeg and cloves)

- coarse foods such as raw fruits and vegetables, dry toast, grainy cereals and breads, and crunchy snacks

- alcoholic beverages

- extremely hot foods or beverages

Dry Mouth

Dry mouth is a common side-effect of total body irradiation, anti-nausea medications, and antihistamines. If a dry mouth is making eating difficult, try the following:

- Add sauces, gravies, broth and dressings to foods.

- Suck ice chips, popsicles, gum or sugarless hard candies to keep the mouth moist.

- Try including citric acid in your diet to stimulate saliva production (unless you have mouth or throat sores). Citric acid is present in oranges, orange juice, lemons, lemonade and sugarless lemon drops. You can also add lemon to tea, water and soda.

- Drink liquids with your meals.

- Practice good mouth care.

- Ask your dietitian or doctor about commercial saliva substitutes such as Salivart®, Mouth-Kote®, Saliva Substitute®, and Xerolube®.

If you have difficulty eating because of a dry mouth, avoid eating plain meats, bread products, crackers, or dry cake. You should also avoid very hot foods or beverages, as well as alcoholic beverages.

Changes in Taste

Total body irradiation, some chemotherapy drugs, certain pain medications, and some antibiotics can temporarily alter the way food and beverages taste, making some foods unappetizing. To overcome this problem, try the following:

- Eat and drink foods and beverages cold or at room temperature.

- Eat strongly flavored foods such as chocolate, lasagna, spaghetti or bar-bequed foods (unless you also have mouth or throat sores).

- Eat tart or spicy foods (unless you also have mouth or throat sores).

- Select foods that smell appetizing.

- Drink fluids with your meal to rinse away any bad taste.

- Eat protein foods without strong odors, such as poultry, eggs, and dairy products rather than those with strong odors such as beef and fish.

- Use plastic utensils if foods seem to have a metallic taste.

- Add sauces to foods.

- Try eating meat with something sweet, such as cranberry sauce, jelly or applesauce.

- Try experimenting with new seasoning combinations or adding sugar, salt or other flavor to enhance the taste.

Thick Saliva

Thick saliva is sometimes a side effect of total body irradiation. It may also be caused by dehydration. If you are experiencing eating difficulties as a result of thick saliva, try the following:

- Drink club soda (seltzer) or hot tea with lemon.

- Try sucking sugarless sour lemon drops.

- Eat a lighter breakfast if you have mucous build up in the morning, and bigger meals in the afternoon and evening.

- Rinse frequently with a saline solution (one quart water with 1/2 to 3/4 teaspoons salt, and one to two teaspoons baking soda).

- Drink lots of fluids.

- Eat soft, tender foods such as cooked fish and chicken, eggs, noodles, thinned cereals, blenderized fruits and vegetables diluted to a very thin consistency.

- Eat small, frequent meals.

- Drink diluted juices, broth-based soups, and fruit-flavored beverages such as Kool-Aid® or Hi-C®.

- Switch to a liquid diet if the problem is severe.

- Ask your doctor about a medication called Salagen® that may increase your saliva.

Patients with thick saliva should avoid eating meats that require chewing, bread products, gelatin desserts, oily foods, hot cereals, thick cream soups and nectars.

Nausea and Vomiting

Following high-dose chemotherapy or total body irradiation, patients often ex-perience nausea and vomiting. Drugs to control infections such as Bactrim® or Septra®, opioid pain control medications, interferon, and mucous drainage from mouth and sinuses may also cause nausea and vomiting.

If nausea and vomiting are interfering with your ability to eat, try the following:

- Eat small, frequent meals.

- Eat dry crackers or toast, especially before movement, such as getting out of bed.

- Eat cold foods, rather than warm foods, because they tend to have less food odor.

- Eat low-fat foods such as cooked vegetables, canned fruit, baked skinless chicken, sherbet, fruit ice, popsicles, gelatin, pretzels, toast, crackers, vanilla wafers, and angel food cake.

- Drink clear, cool liquids such as carbonated beverages, flavored gelatin, popsicles, and ice cubes made of a favorite liquid.

- Sip liquids slowly through a straw.

- Sip or drink small amounts of liquid frequently throughout the day.

- If you're hospitalized, ask that food trays be brought to you without covers on the plates to avoid being overwhelmed by the smell.

- Request medications to control the nausea if it is severe.

- Keep food solely in kitchen areas and leave the kitchen if you feel queasy.

Patients who are troubled by nausea should avoid cooking areas where smells might be offensive. Spicy, overly sweet, high fat and strong smelling foods should be eliminated from the diet until the nausea subsides. Drinking hot liquids or a lot of liquids with meals can also trigger nausea.

If you are nauseated, avoid lying flat on your back after eating. This can make the problem worse. If you need rest, sit or recline with your head elevated. Avoid perfumes and other strong smelling cosmetics.

Lack of Appetite/Weight Loss

Many transplant patients experience weight loss and lack of appetite for a period of time. Possible causes include total body irradiation, chemotherapy, infection, depression and fatigue. If you have no appetite for food following your transplant try the following:

- Eat small frequent high-calorie meals.

- Drink high-nutrient liquids such as juice or milk instead of low-calorie drinks like coffee, tea or diet soda.

- Eat nutrient-dense high-calorie foods such as cheese, whole milk, cream, whipped cream, sour cream, cottage cheese, ice cream, extra butter or powdered milk, eggs, oil, mayonnaise, peanut butter, wheat germ, nuts, instant breakfast beverages and fruits.

- Use carbohydrate supplements such as Polycose®, protein powders such as Promod® or complete nutrition supplements such as Ensure®, Boost®, Carnation Instant Breakfast® or Sustacal®, provided they have been approved by your dietitian. Nonfat dry milk powder can also be added to casseroles, cooked cereals and mixed dishes.

- Create a pleasant, mealtime atmosphere, e.g. colorful place settings, varied food colors and textures, soft music, enhancing food aromas.

- Engage in light exercise to stimulate your appetite.

- Keep trying to eat (unless you are nauseated). Remember that for now, eating may just be a chore to help you get better, not the pleasure that it was before transplant.

- Address any psychological problems that may be causing the loss of appetite with the help of a psychologist or social worker.

- Ask your doctor about an oral medication called Megace® that may improve your appetite.

Diarrhea

Diarrhea can occur following total body irradiation or high-dose chemotherapy. Some antibiotics and oral medications, such as magnesium salts or metoclo-pramide (Reglan®) can also cause diarrhea. In other cases, diarrhea may be caused by infection or lactose intolerance — an inability to digest the lactose in milk products.

If you are experiencing diarrhea try the following:

- Eat smaller amounts of food at each meal.

- Increase your intake of fluids to prevent dehydration.

- Drink fluids between meals rather than with meals.

- Eat and drink foods and beverages high in potassium and low in fiber such as ripe bananas, potatoes without the skin, tomato juice, Gatorade®, orange juice, peach and pear nectar, baked fish and chicken, ground beef, eggs, well-cooked vegetables (except beans, broccoli, cauliflower and cabbage), canned fruit, rice and white bread.

- Use Lactaid® treated dairy products or low-lactose milk and dairy products.

- While you are having difficulty with diarrhea, avoid eating high-fiber foods such as bran, whole grain cereals and bread, raw vegetables, fruits with skin and seeds, popcorn, nuts and seeds.

- Do not take over-the-counter medications like Imodium® unless approved by your doctor, since these drugs can sometimes make a colon infection worse.

- Avoid foods that can cause gas or cramps such as carbonated beverages, beans, broccoli, cauliflower, cabbage, chewing gum, and highly-spiced foods, as well as foods with rich gravies and sauces.

- Foods that contain caffeine such as tea, coffee, chocolate, colas and other caffeinated soft drinks can also aggravate the problem.

Constipation

Some chemotherapy drugs, opioid pain medications, and anti-nausea medica-tions cause constipation and make a patient less enthused about eating. If you are having difficulty with constipation try the following:

- Increase your fluid intake.

- Drink warm beverages.

- Eat high-fiber foods such as raw fruits and vegetables, whole wheat bread and cereals, dried fruit, dried peas and beans. Be sure you drink plenty of fluids while eating these foods.

- Engage in light exercise.

Ask your doctor about stool softeners or laxatives if the problem persists for more than two days.

Resources
Eating and maintaining your weight is very important after transplant. Most transplant programs have a registered dietician available to help patients manage eating difficulties during treatment. If you continue to have eating difficulties long-term, consult the dietician at your transplant center.

To learn more go to our web site at:

www.bmtinfonet.org/after/eatingproblems

Autologous Stem Cell Transplants: A Handbook for Patients

Chapter Eleven
RELIEVING PAIN

I was given a wonderful little button that allowed me to dispense morphine every five minutes. I pushed it a lot. I don't remember much more about that week — I've blocked it out. It's a fog and I'm glad.

Jim King, five-year transplant survivor

For many people about to undergo an autologous transplant, the prospect of pain is more frightening than any other potential complication. In this chapter we'll examine the type of pain patients may experience and the various drugs used to control it. We'll also discuss some non-drug techniques that can help provide relief.

What is Pain?

Today's pain specialists agree that pain is whatever a patient says it is, whenever, wherever and to whatever degree he says it occurs. The sensation of pain is influenced by physical factors such as tissue damage, and by psychological, social and environmental factors.

A football player who cracks a rib while making a spectacular play, for example, may feel only a twinge of pain during the excitement of the game. When that distraction ends, however, his pain will become more intense.

Two different people with the same amount of tissue damage may experience very different levels of pain. Moreover, each person's body absorbs and processes pain medications differently. Thus, the amount of medication required to ease one person's pain may differ greatly from that required to ease another's pain. In short, pain is a very personal experience requiring a highly individualized response from the medical team.

Pain can be described as acute or chronic. Acute pain, usually due to tissue damage, is shorter in duration and ends once the tissue damage is healed. Most pain experienced by autologous transplant patients is acute pain. The word acute does not mean that the pain is sharper or more uncomfortable. It simply refers to the length of time over which pain occurs. Acute pain lasts days or weeks.

Chronic pain persists over months or years and is caused by irreparable tissue damage, nerve damage, or by unknown causes. Often, chronic pain can only be controlled; its source cannot be eliminated.

How Pain is Experienced

The pain experienced by patients undergoing an autologous transplant is usually caused by temporary inflammation of tissues or nerves. The problem may result from chemotherapy, radiation, infection, veno-occlusive disease or medications the patient is taking.

Sensors at the tissue or nerve site detect the physical damage and transmit distress signals to the brain.

Suffering is the person's response to those pain signals. The degree of suffering varies greatly according to the person's emotional and physical condition at the time pain is experienced. Fatigue, depression, anxiety, physical weakness, memories of how well the patient (or doctor) managed the pain in the past and fears about the cause of the pain can increase the suffering associated with pain.

Blocking Pain Signals

The sensation of pain is relieved by blocking the pain signals as they travel from the site of the injury to the brain. Blocking is accomplished through the use of drugs, or through a combination of drug and non-drug therapies.

The most commonly used pain medications for transplant patients are opioids, also known as narcotics. Opioids include drugs such as morphine and hydromorphone (Dilaudid®). Non-opioid drugs such as aspirin, Motrin® and Tylenol® are often not strong enough to provide sufficient pain relief, and may have side effects that can cause problems for transplant patients.

At some transplant centers, non-drug therapies have been combined successfully with pain medications to enhance relief. They include massage, application of heat or cold to the affected area, exercise, relaxation, visualization, hypnosis and distraction. These techniques are discussed later in this chapter.

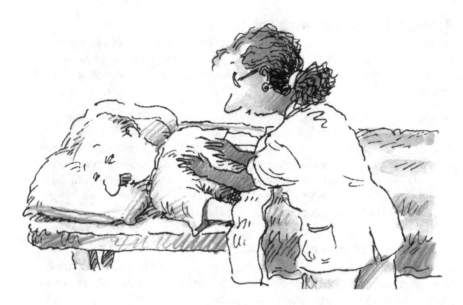

Knowing What to Expect

Information is the cornerstone of any good pain management program. Although the type and amount of pain experienced during a transplant varies from patient to patient, it is helpful to know in advance what type of pain is normal, the cause of the pain, how long it is likely to last, and what will be done to relieve it. If you know approximately when pain will end, it can be tolerated much better than if you think it will go on forever.

It helps to think about painful procedures in sections. A bone marrow aspirate, for example, may take twenty minutes to perform, but the painful part lasts only two minutes, not twenty. Understanding that fact can relieve some of the anxiety associated with the medical procedure. Most of us believe we can tolerate two minutes of pain more easily than twenty minutes of discomfort.

Ask your doctor or nurse to use words other than pain or hurt to describe the sensations you may feel during and after medical procedures. Pain and hurt mean different things to different people. If your doctor does not use a more precise description, you may imagine that the sensation will be much more uncomfortable than it actually is. Words like pressure, stinging, burning, and dull ache convey a much better image of what patients will feel than "pain." When the sensation occurs, you will know that it's expected, and that you're doing okay.

Talking With Children About Pain

The language chosen to describe potentially painful procedures to children should be age-appropriate. Children often misinterpret common medical terms that adults take for granted. For example, some children confuse "bone marrow" with "bow and arrow."

Young children may think that pain is a punishment for bad behavior, and this issue should be clarified before the discomfort begins. Allow children to rehearse painful procedures in advance, or to practice the procedure on dolls or adults. It's best to break the procedure into small steps, moving on to the next step only after the child's anxiety about the first step has been relieved. Combining rehearsals with relaxation and imagery can be a very effective way to desensitize children to uncomfortable procedures.

Identifying the Cause of Pain

In order to properly treat pain, its cause must be identified. Most pain has a physical cause that can either be seen by a physician or deduced based on the patient's history and description of the pain.

Sometimes a physical cause for the pain is not readily apparent. This does not mean that the pain is any less real or less urgent to relieve. Pain experts agree that when a patient says that he is experiencing pain, it's important to take that complaint seriously and attempt to relieve it, whether or not a physical cause is apparent.

Patients can help their physicians properly identify the cause of pain by being very specific about the description, intensity, location and frequency of the pain.

- Rate the pain on a scale of 0-10 (0=no pain, 10=worst pain). Is it mild, moderate or severe?

- Is it sharp or a dull ache? Does it throb? Is there a burning or itching sensation associated with it?

- Is it constant or intermittent? If it's intermittent, how often does it occur? How long does it last?

- When did it begin?

- Do certain actions or motions such as lying down or taking a deep breath make the pain better or worse?

The more information the physician has about the pain, the more likely she will be able to identify and treat both the cause and symptoms properly.

Notify your physician or nurse about pain as soon as it begins. Pain is easier to relieve in the early stages than after it has become severe. There is no need to endure pain, and no reason to be embarrassed about asking for relief. In fact, refusing pain medication may be harmful. Patients who are gripped by pain are often less willing or able to do important things that are necessary for recovery, such as eating or exercising.

Choosing a Drug and Dosage

The drug chosen to relieve pain will depend on the physical cause of the pain. Opioids are effective in controlling pain from tissue damage, such as mouth sores or skin rashes, but may be less effective in controlling pain associated with nerve irritation, such as that caused by herpes zoster. Anti-depressants and anti-convulsants can help control pain caused by nerve damage.

The dosage of medication required to relieve pain varies considerably among patients. There is nothing wrong with the patient who requires more medication to relieve pain. Each person's body reacts differently to pain medications.

Some drugs are very slow acting but produce long-term pain relief. Others quickly reduce pain but are effective only for a short period of time. A combination of drugs is sometimes used to provide patients with the best relief.

Maintaining Relief

If pain increases, the dosage of a drug needed to relieve the pain may also increase. Some drugs, such as opioids, provide additional pain relief whenever the dosage is increased; others do not.

Increasing the dosage of drugs may increase the risk of side effects. These side effects are usually minor and reversible but you should not increase the dosage or frequency of pain medications without checking with your doctor.

While in the hospital or clinic, nurses may administer pain medications or you may be given a Patient Controlled Analgesia machine or PCA, which allows you to administer your own pain medication, up to safe limit, as needed. The PCA can be adjusted to dispense pain medication during periods when you are sleeping. Pain relief may also be administered by a pain patch applied to the skin which delivers narcotics continuously for three days.

Patients who continue to require pain medication after leaving the hospital or clinic often find that a system of reminders helps ensure that pain medications are taken regularly. Placing each day's dosage of drugs in a separate container (most pharmacies sell weekly compartmentalized containers for this purpose), keeping a chart of when each drug is to be taken and making a note after each drug is taken, helps ensure that medications are taken on schedule.

Pain Experienced by Autologous Transplant Patients

Each person's transplant experience is unique. Some people experience only mild discomfort and need only small amounts of pain medication. Others experience more significant pain and require more medication to control it.

Painful mouth sores are a frequent side effect of autologous transplantation. Pain medications such as Lidocaine® can be used like a mouth wash to control the discomfort. In many cases, an opioid such as morphine is given to provide additional relief.

High-dose chemotherapy and radiation can cause skin sores. Opioids are typically used to control the pain. If a burning sensation accompanies the pain, aloe vera gel (not with an alcohol base), Eucerin® or Silvaderm/Lidocaine® cream may be applied directly to the skin.

Certain medical procedures can cause temporary discomfort. A bone marrow aspirate is a good example. In this procedure, a needle is inserted into the rear of the hip bone to withdraw a tiny sample of bone marrow. While the area around the bone can be numbed, it's not possible to numb the bone itself. An uncomfortable scraping sensation and pressure are common with bone marrow aspirates.

Anxiety about the procedure can be reduced by pre-medicating the patient with a small amount of Versed® or Ativan® to relax him and a small dose of opioid to help pain. Don't be embarrassed to ask for pre-medication to ease your anxiety if you're fearful about a bone marrow aspirate.

Other medical procedures that may cause discomfort include lumbar punctures (spinal taps), placement of catheters and rarely, lung biopsies. Opioids are usually effective in relieving pain associated with these procedures.

Children, in particular, may find certain medical procedures distressing. For some, pre-medication helps relieve their anxiety. For others, however, additional sedation is required. A number of centers briefly sedate patients with powerful, short-term general anesthetics, in addition to local anesthetics, so that the patient is not fully conscious while the procedure is taking place. This technique, called conscious sedation, requires an anesthesiologist and more elaborate preparation such as withholding food and drink for six to seven hours prior to the procedure. If you are anxious about painful medical procedures, inquire about of this technique.

Infections may cause mild, moderate or severe pain. Opioids are not effective in eliminating infection-related pain, but can help control the pain while the antibiotic or anti-fungal drug begins to work. If infection develops after a patient is discharged from the hospital or clinic, he may need to be hospitalized for several days to quickly bring the infection and pain under control.

Growth factors used to speed the recovery of a patient's bone marrow after transplant can cause mild to moderate bone pain, muscle pain and/or headaches. In most cases, the pain can be controlled with acetaminophen and usually ends when the patient stops taking these drugs. If the pain is severe, opioids may be used to relieve it.

Fear of Addiction

One of the biggest barriers to providing patients with adequate pain relief is the erroneous belief by much of the public, and some medical professionals, that taking opioid pain medications will lead to drug addiction. Thus, some patients opt to put up with pain rather than ask for pain medication, and some physicians who are inexperienced in modern pain control techniques prescribe inadequate dosages of opioids to relieve pain. Unless a patient has a history of drug or alcohol addiction, he is unlikely to become addicted to pain medications during transplant.

What if Pain Continues?

Since pain relief must be tailored to each individual's needs, it may take some time before the appropriate type and level of pain medication can be determined. You can help your doctor by providing feedback on how well the pain medications are working. Has the medication provided any relief at all? Does the drug wear off before you're scheduled to take the next dosage? Are you experiencing any side effects such as drowsiness, nervousness, nausea, itching or constipation?

When you are given pain medication, ask when you can expect it to take effect. While you're waiting for it to work, try to find a distraction from the pain. If the drug fails to relieve the pain when expected, notify your doctor or nurse. He will adjust the dosage or change your prescription until pain relief is achieved.

If you feel you are not receiving adequate pain relief, talk to your doctor or ask a family member to raise this problem with the doctors and nurses. Spouses, parents and other caregivers can be very effective advocates for patient pain relief, particularly when a patient is too exhausted or embarrassed to seek help on his own.

Non-Drug Pain Control Techniques

Olympic athletes do it. Football stars do it. In fact everyone, at some time or another, has relied on non-drug pain control methods to relieve discomfort.

When a child falls and bruises himself, a parent may show him an interesting toy to take his attention away from the pain. Women preparing for childbirth often take prenatal classes that teach them how to use breathing exercises to relieve pain during labor and delivery. Heat, cold, immobilization, or physical therapy is commonly used by athletes to relieve pain caused by sports injuries.

While drugs are the primary source of pain relief for transplant patients, non-drug therapies can enhance pain relief. Non-drug pain control techniques are not a substitute for effective pain medications, but are important tools that can help patients better manage their pain.

Several non-drug therapies are available to patients, including positive coping statements, distraction, relaxation, imagery, hypnosis, application of heat or cold to the affected area, massage, and exercise.

Positive Coping Statements

Fear and a feeling of helplessness are common among transplant patients. Not only has a powerful disease taken control of their body, but they are forced to rely on a team of complete strangers to save their life. Anger and frustration over this lack of control can lead to anxiety and depression, which in turn can make it more difficult to tolerate pain.

Although these negative thoughts and feelings are normal, you can often exercise some control over them with positive coping statements. Focus on the various things you can do rather than those that you can't do. Try to take encouragement from even small accomplishments, or find something positive in each experience.

For example, if you're discouraged because the days of treatment seem to be passing slowly, try focusing on the fact that you have already successfully made it through several days, and that you are moving closer to the day of full recovery. If you experience some backsliding, e.g., your blood counts go down or your body is not responding to certain medications, explain to yourself that temporary setbacks are normal and not a cause for alarm. Think about the progress you have made overall since starting your treatment and try not to measure each day against the successes of a prior day.

Some patients find that repeating encouraging phrases like prayers, or the words 'I am coping well,' help.

> "I had a friend — an older gentleman — who came to my house before the transplant. He was 6'-4", had a tall crop of white hair, wore cowboy boots, lean jeans and a rope tie. He said he was going to help me relax and keep the pain from my mind. He taught me several relaxation techniques. I was always able to call him and he'd give me some key words or phrases that helped me start relaxing until the medications arrived or until I stopped panicking."

If it is difficult to find something positive in each day's experience, ask the hospital social worker, pastoral counselor, psychologist or psychiatry staff for help. Often they can suggest ways to cope with your frustrations and refocus your attention on more positive thoughts.

Distraction

Distraction is probably the most familiar non-drug pain control technique. Watching a movie, listening to soothing music, or talking with visitors diverts our attention from discomfort and focuses it on a more pleasurable experience.

Before your transplant, think about the kinds of activities that will help pass the time and provide a distraction from worry and pain. Set aside recordings of music or stories, movies (with uncomplicated plots), books (simple stories or picture books may be all you can handle), and video or family games that you enjoy. Keep in mind that you'll often be groggy, your attention span will be shorter, and your coordination will be temporarily diminished while you're taking medication. Thus, you may not be able to handle the more complicated hobbies or activities you normally enjoy until later.

You may find that conversations with family members or friends are the most helpful distraction from pain. Having a caregiver read to you or simply listening to conversations among visitors can be pleasant.

Storytelling is an excellent distraction for children. Letting the child tell the story with you works best, but listening to stories can be helpful as well. Art projects also work well with children who are usually less inhibited than adults about testing their artistic talents and ideas.

Relaxation and Imagery

Relaxation and imagery are two commonly used techniques to relieve anxiety and pain. Relaxation involves a series of muscle tensing and relaxing exercises or focused breathing exercises that are designed to induce a sense of calm in the body.

Relaxation is most effective when combined with imagery. Imagery involves thinking of a pleasant, safe, relaxing or exciting place or activity that brings you happiness. Exploring this place or activity in your mind in great detail can help induce a sense of calm.

> "When I began to panic or experience discomfort, I'd close my eyes and concentrate on my own breathing until all I could hear was my breathing and heartbeat. Then I'd picture my toes and try to put them to sleep, and work my way up my legs, thighs, hips, arms, and hands until I felt very heavy. Once I achieved that heaviness, I'd try to picture a place I'd like to be and concentrate on the details. I pictured myself as sixteen-years-old, wearing a white gauzy dress, sitting with my dog on my favorite patchwork quilt in a forest glen, with the rays of the sun coming through the trees. My long hair would be blowing in the breeze, and it felt good. After that, I would be calm."

Relaxation and imagery techniques are easy to learn, but they take an initial investment of time, concentration and practice to master. They're most effective if learned in advance of your transplant when you're better able to concentrate.

Depending on the complexity of the relaxation technique and whether you're learning it alone or with guidance, it may require as much as one to two weeks of practice before you can use it effectively. Experiment with several methods until you find one that's right for you and then stick with it. Practice at least twice daily for five to ten minutes.

Hypnosis

Hypnosis is often used by therapists in conjunction with distraction and imagery to help patients change the way they experience pain, time, sensations of heat, cold and touch, and a sense of connection to one's body. Hypnosis may enable a patient to think about the painful area of his body as a separate, unconnected part, or shorten his perception of how long the painful experience lasts.

A skilled therapist will individualize the use of hypnosis to help each person develop those techniques that work best for him. Hypnosis is best taught by an experienced clinician who knows a variety of other approaches to pain management as well.

Some people have an easier time using hypnosis than others. Children appear to be more hypnotizable than adults since they are more willing to engage in fantasy. To locate a therapist in your area who is skilled in hypnosis, contact the department of behavioral medicine at a cancer center near you.

Physical Stimulation

Suffering is triggered by pain signals transmitted through the nervous system and spinal cord to the brain. One way to dull these pain signals is to provide a different, competing physical sensation.

Applying heat or cold to painful areas often masks pain signals and reduces suffering. Ice packs, however, should not be used for six months on skin that has been irradiated. Massage can also provide a soothing sensation that competes with pain signals.

Some patients find exercise a potent pain reliever:

> "I developed a case of shingles after my transplant. I continued to
> have discomfort long after the sores had healed. I tried everything
> to control the pain including acupuncture and pain pills. Nothing
> worked. Finally, I began to work out at the gym seven days a week.
> That turned out to be the best pain relief of all."

Learning to Use the Techniques

Learning non-drug pain control techniques before pain becomes intolerable is the key to using them successfully. Many hospitals with cancer programs offer classes that teach relaxation and imagery skills, or provide individual instruction and assistance.

While non-drug pain control techniques will not cure your disease or take the place of pain medications, they can give you a greater sense of control over your body and help make the healing process more tolerable.

Conclusion

After your transplant, don't hesitate to seek the help of a pain specialist if you feel your local physician is not taking your complaints of pain seriously or is unable to prescribe adequate pain medication. Most physicians have not received specialized training in pain control and some are more experienced than others in this rapidly evolving area of medicine.

Many universities and large hospitals now have special pain control programs with experts in both drug and non-drug pain control techniques who may be able to help you. To find a pain control specialist consult the American Pain Foundation at www.painfoundation.org or phone 888-615-PAIN (7246).

To learn more go to our web site at:

www.bmtinfonet.org/webcast and scroll down to find the webcast on managing pain.

Autologous Stem Cell Transplants: A Handbook for Patients

Chapter Twelve
CAREGIVING

Pamper not only the patient, but the caregiver as well. Caregivers need mail, home-cooked meals, a gift certificate to their favorite store, bath gel, something they would never get themselves (like music, a book, candy, a gourmet candy bar) — something to brighten their day and make them feel special. Even if you just send a $10 check with a note that says, 'Thought you could use a little extra something' — these things make a big difference. Long after the transplant, regardless of whether it's successful or not, memories of the experience will linger with the caregiver. Out of the blue, write or call. It's important that caregivers know you're still thinking of them.

Sarah Routman, mother of a 22-month-old transplant patient

An autologous transplant is a very difficult experience for patients and family members alike. As everyone's attention focuses on saving the patient's life, the needs of one of the patient's most important partners — the family member or friend who is the primary caregiver — are often underestimated.

Caring for a transplant patient is physically challenging and emotionally draining. Watching as a loved one undergoes difficult medical procedures taxes even the most optimistic and healthy caregiver. Helping other family members cope with the experience adds to the burden.

Most caregivers agree on one thing: you must take care of yourself to be a good giver of care. In this chapter, the role of the primary caregiver will be discussed. Much of the information is from those who have been a caregiver for a transplant patient. They will share their experiences, what they feel they did well and what they could have done better. (Additional issues faced by parents who are caregivers for pediatric patients are discussed in Chapter Six, When Your Child Needs a Transplant.)

Taking Time to Recharge

In order to provide the best possible care for the patient, caregivers need to take time off for themselves to recharge. There are many things that can be done to relieve the stress of caregiving, get a clear head and find a little bit of perspective. Whether you choose to go for a walk, take in a movie, visit with friends, or just nap, taking time for yourself is essential, say former caregivers.

> "Even though you may not want to or think you need to, getting away from the caregiving world for even half an hour is important. One person, even a workaholic, can't handle this situation alone."

> "You're going to feel tired, frustrated, even annoyed at your loved one sometimes, and that's OK. It's a very stressful time for every- one and you are only human. Even though you love the person going through the transplant, there will be days when you are just plain tired of the hospital, the disease and the treatment. Try to take some time for yourself. Go for a walk outside. Get away from the hospital if just for a few minutes. Write in a journal, read a book, work on a project (I put photos in an album). You are not being selfish. You have to take time for yourself in order to really help your loved one."

The need to take time for yourself doesn't end when the treatment is over and the patient returns home. At home, the caregiver must assume many tasks that were handled by nurses in the hospital or clinic. It is critical to pace your- self, say caregivers, because you may be giving care intensively for a long time.

> "When my wife came home from the hospital, caring for her was even harder than it was while she was hospitalized. I no longer had nurses and doctors on hand to monitor her, and I had to be con- stantly vigilant to detect problems. That was a lot of stress. During times when the patient is not in danger, try to take a few days away for yourself. You will be under a lot of stress for the long-haul, and you need to get some relief."

Some caregivers have found that classes on how to care for chronically ill patients, offered at some hospitals or health agencies, help ease the strain.

> "The transplant center instructed me on things specific to trans- plant patients, like how to take care of the catheter. But courses for caregivers offered at our local hospital were also helpful. They taught the basics of caring for chronically ill patients — like how to help them without disrupting the household, how to help them walk without injuring yourself, etc. It was basic information that would be covered in a nursing assistance course."

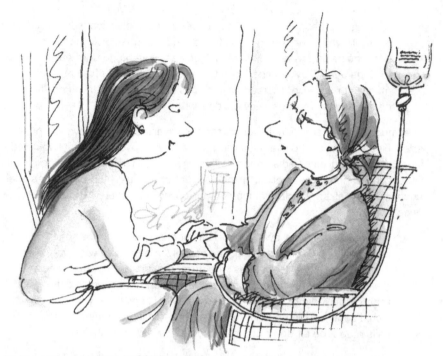

Taking Care of Physical Well Being

A caregiver is only effective if he or she is in good physical condition. Constantly overdoing it can backfire. "Eat well balanced meals, exercise and sleep when you can," one caregiver advises. "You need to stay well in order to take proper care of the patient."

> "Learn, develop and practice good self-care skills prior to the transplant. Once the transplant begins, your primary attention will be on the patient, and you'll have little time or energy left to learn these skills."

> "I knew from the start I was in for a long haul and had to take care of myself. I set 11 pm as my curfew and let my wife know I had to leave the hospital then so I could sleep and come back in the morning refreshed. I pretty much stuck to that except for those nights when things weren't going well. When I stayed overnight at the hospital, I really paid for it for the next two to three days."

Managing Feelings

One of the complexities of being a caregiver is that it's not neutral — caregivers are taking care of patients about whom they care deeply. People who have done it stress the importance of having a forum for processing feelings and fears apart from the patient. "Don't count on the patient to understand your emotional needs," says one caregiver. "Lean on others for support."

"Don't get so caught up worrying about everyone else that you don't deal with your own feelings and fears. Find a counselor or someone who understands what you are going through and talk your feelings out. Allow yourself to cry. I didn't do this, and after several months of anxiety, I started having physical symptoms. If you don't deal with your feelings, they will deal with you."

The importance of emotional support for caregivers cannot be over-emphasized. Find someone who is a good listener, who will let you talk about your feelings. Some caregivers find a special friend or small circle of friends works well. Others find the families of other transplant patients most helpful. Professional counseling or talks with clergy helped many caregivers deal with the experience.

"It helps to have your own network of friends whose number one concern is how you are doing. The caregiver is so busy worrying about what the patient needs, she often doesn't recognize her own feelings. I had a few family members and friends who would contact me periodically to see how I was doing. I kept a diary and would send it to them, and they'd call or write in response. Their calls made me sit down and think about how I was really feeling."

"I frequently talked with other families on the transplant unit. They were in as much pain as I was and understood what I was going through. We all helped each other. We were one big family."

"Seek counseling and the help of a spiritual advisor before the transplant begins. This experience changed my belief system on a very deep level and in ways I could not have predicted. I was grateful to have an already established channel for expressing and discussing these changes."

BMT InfoNet can link caregivers with others who have been through the experience. Phone 888-597-7674 or visit www.bmtinfonet.org and click on "Patients & Families" and then select "Talk to a Survivor or Family Member" from the drop down list.

Accepting Help

Planning for the long haul includes inviting and accepting help from others. Many people assume that the transplant is simply their own problem to manage. Yet taking care of a very sick patient and managing the usual household and work chores is more than most people can handle.

Extended family members and friends often truly want to help, but don't know what would be most appreciated. Figure out what people are good at and give them jobs that suit their temperament and skills. If someone enjoys physical activity, let that friend cut the grass. Good cooks can prepare meals. Parents of your children's friends can help shuttle them to school and after school activities. It all helps. "Develop a strong network of support before the transplant," advises a former caregiver. "This will free you up to focus on the patient's needs."

> "One of the hardest things for both of us to learn was to let other people help us. We weren't used to having other people do things for us. We always assumed there would have to be a payback. But people would take the kids shopping for school clothes, take them to the show, etc. and refuse money when I offered it to them. Finally we had to accept the fact that we could never repay everyone for their kindness. There were too many people helping us for that. It made a big change in our lives to realize how many friends we really had."

Being the Patient's Advocate

Part of being the patient's caregiver is being his advocate. Caregivers know information about the patient that doctors and nurses may not have. You may know, for example, how best to get your child to do unpleasant tasks. If you are caring for an adult patient, you may know that the patient will be reluctant to ask for pain relief before the pain is severe and more difficult to control.

Although the transplant team works hard to provide the best care for patients, they may not always pick up patient distress signals as easily as a caregiver who knows the patient well. It comforts patients to know that their caregiver is looking out for their well-being only, and is not distracted by the needs of other patients.

> "I saw my job as a gatekeeper — keeping track of details, asking questions, being an advocate for my wife with the medical staff and taking care of her emotional and physical needs. I was present at all the medical consultations and made sure I paid attention to details like whether she was receiving proper medicines. When visitors came I managed them, depending on whether or not my wife wanted to see them."

> "I made a point of becoming very well informed about the transplant process. I felt strongly that I was an advocate for my husband, and in order to be taken seriously and to get the best care for him, I had to be knowledgeable. At the same time, I worked hard to ignore statistics. They're useful for scientists, but not patients. A person cannot be 20% alive and 80% dead, so it's pointless to get hung up on the numbers."

Getting Information

Although getting information on a daily basis from the patient's doctor is important, it's sometimes hard to accomplish. Find out when the doctors make their rounds each day so you can be there to ask questions. Stop the doctor at any time when you don't understand what she's saying, and ask her to explain it again. If you are unable to be present when the doctor visits the patient, find out when you can contact her by phone or visit in person.

One family who had multiple caregivers left a journal with the patient. All caregivers wrote in it daily about the patient's medical care, other important details, and feelings. Some people even tape recorded or videotaped meetings with doctors to help them keep track of important information.

> "Keep a diary and carry it with you. I would write down everything in it — doctors' instructions, names, phone numbers, maps, etc. One day starts to blend into the next and it becomes impossible to remember everything without taking notes."

Both patients and caregivers are often unprepared for the fact that the physicians rotate off duty each month. Find out when doctors rotate, so you can debrief the doctor who is leaving, get some information about the doctor who is about to assume your loved one's care, and prepare the patient for the change, advise caregivers.

Flexibility and Patience: Essential Components

As it is with many things in life, each transplant evolves in its own way. There is no way to predict how someone's course will unfold. The caregiver needs to be prepared for ups and downs during the patient's treatment and recovery. Complications occur, and recovery sometimes takes longer than expected. After the patient returns home, there can be setbacks. It's common for transplant patients to develop infections and other complications that may require them to be admitted to the hospital.

> "Plan all you can, but expect the unexpected. Plan to be more tired than you can possibly imagine. Take things one day at a time or, if necessary, one hour at a time and hang in there."

> "I tried to say the serenity prayer every day. 'God, grant me the serenity to accept things I cannot change, courage to change the things I can, and the wisdom to know the difference.' "

Keeping a Sense of Humor

Many caregivers say that maintaining a sense of humor, despite the difficulties, helped them and the patient cope.

> "Through all the tears, we managed to find a lot of humor, which kept us all sane. Sometimes things that seem so traumatic at the time can really strike you funny in retrospect. For example, when my sister was having her chemotherapy, the nurses suggested

she shave off her hair, rather than let it fall out. My dad wanted to take pictures of it, and we really argued with him about it — it was so upsetting at the time. But a few days later, when the pictures came back, we all had a good laugh. We couldn't believe we'd been fighting over hair, when there were so many bigger issues at stake."

"When my husband visited my daughter, he always brought a gift. Once he brought in a big, silly, hot pink floppy hat. She wore it and a pair of pig slippers when she walked in the hallway. It gave every one, including the other patients, a lift — something to smile about."

"I would rent funny movies or read funny books to my wife. I also found it helpful to share humorous moments with visitors and friends. The transplant was very scary for our friends. My wife and I were in deep denial as we went through it, but our friends understood the severity of the situation. It made it easier for them to call or visit if we could share some humorous moments with them."

"Pray, cry and talk when you need to, but also keep a positive attitude. During my husband's recovery, we played a lot of cards, talked about all the fun we'd had, and all the fun we were going to have once he was well."

Relaying Information to Others

One task many caregivers find difficult is keeping family and friends informed about the patient's progress. Relying on friends to help with this task eases the burden. So does relying on technology. One woman set up a communication network in advance with family, co-workers and friends.

"It was really draining to get information to all the people who cared. After working all day and being at the hospital, it takes all your energy just to exist some days. My wife and I shared details with four or five close friends who we knew would be a great source of support. For the rest, I recorded a more general message each day on our answering machine."

"I sent a summary of the week's events to family and friends each Saturday night. I began writing in a journal the day my wife went into the hospital. I spent a half hour to one hour each day recording events and our feelings. Initially I did it so my wife would have a record of what happened to her. But it became the way I organized my thoughts, sorted out feelings, and communicated with loved ones. I've continued journaling even to this day."

"My friend's caregiver set up a permanent e-mail list. Each week she sent the entire list an update, including any suggestions she had for supporting the patient at whatever stage she was at in the process."

Online resources like CaringBridge.org or LotsaHelpingHands.org are an excellent way to keep family and friends updated on the patient's progress.

Know Your Role

Caring for an adult who is undergoing an autologous transplant is emotionally trying and physically exhausting. Not only does the caregiver have to juggle the needs of the patient, his own needs, and those of family members, but many must do it without help from the person with whom he normally shares these responsibilities — the patient.

"I think it's tougher for the caregiver than the patient. The patient can stay focused on getting well, but you also have your normal day-to-day stuff like work, children, bills and other family members to deal with. It's a lot of stress."

To complicate matters, the patient and caregiver may have different ideas about the caregiver's role. The caregiver may feel he has to become a medical expert to properly care for the patient, when in reality, what the patient may want most is emotional support.

"Find out what the patient expects from you. My husband just wanted me there, not to entertain him, but for the feeling of companionship, and to give support and comfort during the long recovery process."

"It helps to follow the cues from the patient. Do as little or as much as he wants you to do. Help the patient maintain his dignity by letting him take the lead."

Walking the thin line between being an understanding caregiver and wanting the patient to take a more active role in his recovery can be difficult. Sometimes caregivers feel that the patient should be making more progress, but don't know how hard to push the issue.

"Be patient, but also feel your way into becoming more assertive with the patient. I always felt I shouldn't say certain things to my husband, but then I started feeling depressed and isolated. I waited too long to tell him simple things, like he had enough strength to take out the garbage. He became extremely depressed and dependent on me. That was very hard, but eventually we worked things out."

"Getting the patient to bathe, eat, exercise and take medications is not always easy. Sometimes you have to be stern with instructions. Learn to be patient, but kindly persistent. A good caregiver is not a softy."

Changing Relationships

Being the caregiver for an adult, particularly a spouse, who is recovering from transplant can dramatically alter your relationship — at least for a time. The physical and emotional trauma experienced by both the patient and caregiver is often expressed as anger, irritability or depression. In most cases, the problems resolve over time and some eventually share a closer relationship with their spouse. For others, the changes remain for a long time.

"My husband became very grouchy, impatient and irritable. He expected a lot from me all the time. It was often hard to be patient with him."

"I had to take over all of his responsibilities — paying bills, yard work, etc. Instead of being an equal partner, it was like having another child to worry about. I felt like I'd lost the man I married and just wanted him back."

"We seem to have permanently traded roles. He used to be the more relaxed, practical conscientious partner. Now I have to constantly remind him not to get upset over little things and to be more positive. He experienced some memory loss, and it constantly irritates me that he can't remember things that are important to us. I hate the part of me that feels that way and I haven't told him how I feel because it sounds so ungrateful — I might have lost him completely. Still, between his personality change and my irritation at his memory loss, I sometimes feel like I've lost part of him and myself."

"The changes we've noticed are for the better. We made it through one of the most difficult things a couple can go through. It has changed our perspective and led us to make a number of positive changes in our lives. Which is not to say that we don't still fight about nothing from time to time, but rather that our fighting is half-hearted, as though we know it's nothing."

Helping Children Cope

Children of transplant patients share the trauma of their parent's illness and treatment. Depending on their age, they may express their fears in a number of different ways. Some become depressed. Others have behavioral problems, difficulties at school, or begin to regress. Still others may worry that they caused or will catch the disease.

For most children, just being separated from their parent for a long period of time is very distressing. Being open and honest with children about the parent's disease and treatment, and allowing them to express their questions and concerns is essential to helping them cope with the experience.

> "Our three children, ages two, seven, and eleven, had all kinds of problems. The stress of knowing their mother might not live was overwhelming. I tried to help them by talking with them, over and over again, about my wife's illness. I made sure they understood that there are no stupid questions or feelings."

> "My sister had four children at home, ages seven months to twelve years. They were cared for by their grandmother while their mother was in a hospital 200 miles away. To help the kids cope, my brother arranged for the use of a video phone — one at the hospital and one at home. That helped my sister and the kids tremendously."

> "My 13-year-old son became very depressed while his father was undergoing a transplant out of town. In addition to getting him some professional help, I sent him to visit his father over Spring break. It helped him to see his father alive and progressing."

> "A big concern expressed by our six-year-old daughter was that her mom was going to be bald. We took control of the situation by first taking her to the hospital several times before the transplant to see other people and children who were bald. We then made it a family outing with friends and a movie camera when my wife went to the hair dresser and had her hair buzzed army-style. Our daughter accepted the baldness well and even asked to take her mom to school for 'show and tell'. She was very proud of her bald mom, and my wife went with no reservations."

Coming Home

Everyone looks forward to leaving the hospital or ending the daily visits to the outpatient clinic. Many, however, are unprepared for the fact that for the first months, life at home will not be normal.

In many ways, caring for a transplant patient at home is more difficult than assisting with his care while in the hospital or outpatient clinic. Medications must be administered, catheters must be carefully cleaned, special diets may have to be followed and infection precautions must be adhered to — all without the help of a readily available nursing staff.

The early weeks and months are often a confusing and stressful time for families. This is a time when you may experience burn-out. Your loved one has survived the rigors of the treatment and you should be happy, but the difficulties are far from over. There are frequent clinic visits, sometimes a hospitalization, and ongoing caregiving responsibilities. Support systems may begin to fall apart as family and friends mistakenly think that life is now back to normal.

> "Picking up the pieces is not easy. For months I felt like I was on autopilot. I forgot how to sleep and constantly felt like I was dragging. There didn't seem to be enough hours in the day or energy in me to take care of everyone's needs. After ten months I wondered, 'When will this be over?' "

It helps to let friends and family members know how they can help. Although some may not be as understanding as you'd like, others will be glad for the opportunity to help and thankful that you are explicit about what you need.

Conclusion

Happily, most people who survive an autologous transplant report that it was worth the difficulties. Caregivers survive, too, although probably changed from the people they were before the experience.

> "Some good came out of this experience, aside from the fact that my daughter is alive. It helped everyone think about what was important in life."

> "I learned a lot about being a caretaker for a seriously ill family member. It has made me (a doctor) and my wife (a nurse) better caretakers for our patients."

Perhaps this three-and-a-half-year-old survivor said it best to his mom about the importance of caregivers:

> "On the first anniversary of his transplant, I told him it was time to visit the clinic again and he asked, 'Why?'

> I said, 'Everyone who took care of you wants to see you and besides, we should thank the doctors for making you better.'

> He looked at me and said, 'No mommy, you made me better.' "

To learn more go to our web site at:

www.bmtinfonet.org/before/caregivers

Chapter Thirteen

SEXUALITY AFTER TRANSPLANT

No one ever mentioned that my sex life might be affected by transplant. It wouldn't have changed my decision to have a transplant, but it sure would have prepared me better for what to expect and what to do about it.

Robert W, 12-year transplant survivor

It's the elephant in the room: sexual difficulties after transplant. No one talks about it upfront, especially when life and death matters are of primary concern.

Although pop culture is full of sexy images and dialogue, frank and honest discussion about sex is not something that is encouraged. Many people feel embarrassed to even bring it up with their doctor and physicians are equally uncomfortable about discussing it with patients. Hence, the topic is not addressed and patients suffer in silence.

But changes in sexuality after transplant are common and knowing what to expect and how to deal with these changes can ease distress between partners.

Not everyone experiences changes in sexuality after transplant. However, in one study by Syrjala et al, 46% percent of men and 80% percent of women reported lower sexual activity and sexual function five years after transplant than those who have not had a transplant. Women who resumed sexual relations during the first year after transplant had less difficulty later than those who did not.

Changes in sexuality come as a surprise for both patient and partner alike. Fortunately, if sexual difficulties do arise there are several things you can try to remedy the situation and make sexual relationships pleasurable once again.

Talking openly with your partner about any changes in desire, arousal or sexual satisfaction that you are experiencing is important. You will need to work together to address the problem, and communicating about these issues will help you develop a plan. The solution may mean changing the way you seek and enjoy intimate relations. A consultation with a trained sex therapist can be helpful in identifying ways to regain intimacy.

What Causes the Change?

Both radiation and chemotherapy can impact sexual function after transplant. Some anti-depressants and pain medicines can also impact sexual activity.

Males

Men who undergo total body irradiation (TBI) may experience damage to the small blood vessels in the penis. This can make it difficult to achieve an erection. Radiation and some types of high-dose chemotherapy can cause nerve damage and reduced testosterone levels which can impact desire.

Difficulty achieving an erection can be treated by medications such as Viagra®, Cialis® or Levitra®. These drugs relax smooth muscle cells that let blood flow into the penis. However, they don't work as well if nerves have been damaged and they do not increase desire.

Injections of drugs such as Caverject® and Edex® can help men achieve erections. Vacuum devices, although cumbersome, are also very helpful.

Talk with your doctor about whether these or other therapies, such as surgical implants, are appropriate for you.

Most men recover normal testosterone levels between six months and two years after transplant. For those who continue to have low or low-normal testosterone levels, testosterone replacement can help. Skin patches, injections and topical gels are the usual methods of delivery.

Females

Radiation and high-dose chemotherapy usually cause premature ovarian failure. Ovarian failure reduces the ability of the vagina to stretch, and reduces the lubricating fluid in the vagina. The vaginal skin becomes thin and fragile; during intercourse there can be bleeding, soreness or burning. This pain, as well as the usual menopausal symptoms like hot flashes and reduced testosterone, can reduce a woman's desire for sexual intercourse.

Many women report decreased physical arousal, difficulty reaching orgasm or orgasms that are not as intense as they used to be before transplant. Vaginal moisturizers such as Replens®, KY liquibeads® or similar products used regularly can be useful. Water or silicon based lubricants specifically designed for use before intercourse can also help. Some women find that a vaginal dilator improves blood flow to and elasticity of the vagina.

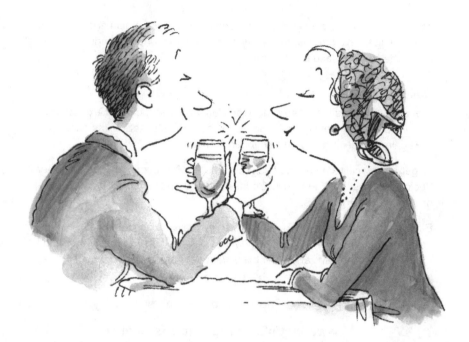

Many women experience early menopause following transplant. Hormone replacement therapy can be useful, although it has been controversial in recent years. A discussion with your doctor about the risks and benefits of this therapy will help you decide whether it is right for you.

One thing is clear: women who resume sexual relationships during their first year after treatment tend to have fewer problems later on. Consulting your doctor and a sex therapist early on can help reduce the likelihood of long-term sexual difficulties.

Psychological Issues

Aside from the physical difficulties created by transplant, psychological issues can also affect a your sexual desire and pleasure. Both you and your partner may worry about infection, particularly if your immune system has not fully recovered. Weight loss or weight gain, scars, temporary hair loss and other physical changes can affect how you feel about your body and sexual appeal.

Some people find that taking it slow and easy helps them transition back into a satisfactory sexual relationship. There are a variety of different techniques you can use to achieve intimacy with a partner. A sex therapist can help you identify some new techniques to try.

The most important thing is to maintain honest, open communication with your partner about what both of you need and can achieve. Don't assume you know what your partner wants. You need to ask. Make a plan and set some ground rules. This can eliminate frustration and misunderstanding and accelerate the road to sexual recovery.

Resources

A booklet available from the American Cancer Society called *Sexuality and Fertility after Cancer*, by Leslie Schover PhD, offers practical insights on how to regain sexual intimacy after cancer therapy.

To get a referral to a certified sex therapist in your area contact the American Society of Sexuality Educators, Counselors and Therapists at www.aasect.org or phone 202-449-1099.

BMT InfoNet offers several webcasts on sexuality after transplant. You can access them at www.bmtinfonet.org/webcast. Scroll down to Sexuality and Intimacy After Transplant and select the webcasts of interest to you.

To learn more go to our web site at:

www.bmtinfonet.org /after/sexuality

Chapter Fourteen
FAMILY PLANNING

Deciding to undergo a transplant was the hardest decision of my life. The odds of survival were not in my favor, and the fact that I would be infertile after the transplant tore me apart. I finally decided I had too much to live for, and too much more to accomplish to give up. I agreed to have the transplant.

Lisa Powell, seven-year transplant survivor

Most, but not all, patients who undergo a blood stem cell transplant will be infertile afterward. The likelihood of infertility depends on the patient's age, gender, sexual maturity, and the type and amount of chemotherapy and/or radiation the patient receives as part of the preparative regimen.

Fortunately, there are options available to couples who wish to have children after transplant. Medically-assisted reproduction techniques such as artificial insemination and in-vitro fertilization are options for women after transplant. Sperm banking before transplant may enable men to have children after transplant. Adoption is another option.

Understanding the options in advance of your transplant will enable you to better plan for children after transplant, and relieve some of the stress associated with the prospect of infertility.

Medically Assisted Reproduction

Couples who wish to bear children after transplant may benefit from recent advances in medically-assisted reproduction technology. While not always successful, assisted reproduction allows women who are infertile to bear children, and men to contribute to the genetic make-up of their child.

Artificial Insemination

Artificial insemination is a procedure in which male sperm are injected into a woman's vagina at the point in her monthly cycle when the mature egg is most likely to have been released into the fallopian tube. If the sperm fertilizes an egg and the resulting embryo implants in the lining of the uterus, a pregnancy begins.

Frozen sperm have been successfully used in artificial insemination. Thus, if you are facing the possibility of infertility after transplant you may wish to bank some of your sperm prior to transplant.

Sperm banking is a relatively simple procedure. Several ejaculates of sperm are collected over a one to three week period and cryopreserved (frozen at very low temperatures) in sterile containers until needed.

Although your sperm count may be lower due to illness or prior chemotherapy, it may still be possible to collect enough sperm for future use.

If your sperm is not frozen prior to transplant, it is still possible for you and your partner to have a child using donor sperm. A donor may be someone you know or sperm from a sperm bank.

In-Vitro Fertilization

Women who are infertile after transplant may be able to carry a child to term with the help of in-vitro fertilization (IVF). IVF enables eggs to be fertilized by male sperm in a laboratory dish. The resulting embryos are then transferred to the woman's uterus. If an embryo implants in the uterine lining a pregnancy begins.

IVF can be done using your own eggs that were collected before transplant or eggs donated by a friend, relative or anonymous donor. Although in-vitro fertilization with donated eggs does not allow you to contribute to the genetic make up of your child, you can carry and nurture a child in your womb during pregnancy, and mother it thereafter.

If you are considering having your own eggs stored prior to your transplant, you should first consult your transplant physician. Some of the drugs used to stimulate egg production might accelerate the disease or otherwise interfere with treatment. In many cases, there may not be sufficient time to complete the procedure before transplant.

New alternatives for preserving fertility before transplant are being explored. Several investigators are exploring whether removing an entire ovary and freezing the outer layer that contains the eggs for future use is a viable option.

For men who have a very low sperm count or low sperm mobility after transplant, intracytoplasmic sperm injection (ICSI) is a potential treatment option.

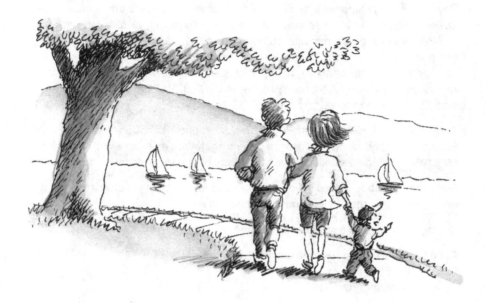

In this procedure, a reproductive specialist inserts a single sperm into the egg to fertilize it. The egg is then implanted in the woman's uterus.

In-vitro fertilization is expensive and insurance may or may not cover the cost. It can take several cycles before in-vitro fertilization is successful, and some couples may not be successful at all. Nonetheless, several transplant survivors have succeeded in becoming pregnant after transplant with the help of in-vitro fertilization.

To learn more about assisted reproduction techniques and the centers that provide these services, contact:

LIVESTRONG/Fertile Hope
866-965-7205
www.fertilehope.org

American Society for Reproductive Medicine
205-978-5000
www.asrm.org

Adoption

People who have been treated for a life-threatening illness may find it difficult to adopt a child in the U.S. through a traditional adoption agency. Most adoption agencies have strict requirements regarding the health history of adopting parents and may deny you because of your prior illness or treatment.

However, it may be possible to arrange for a private domestic adoption. It is advisable to hire a skilled adoption attorney to help you. He or she can prevent you from making costly mistakes, advise you what is allowed under State law, and provide advice on how to publicize your interest in adopting a child. You can find a reputable attorney that specializes in adoption law by contacting the American Academy of Adoption Attorneys at 202-832-2222 or by visiting their web site www.adoptionattorneys.org.

Adopting a child from a country other the U.S. is another option to consider. Each country has its own guidelines regarding the adoptive parents' health history, which may be less restrictive than those of domestic adoption agencies.

Many transplant survivors have successfully adopted children after transplant and are enjoying their role as parent to the fullest.

To learn more about adoption options go to:

Child Welfare Information Gateway
800-394-3366
www.childwelfare.gov

North American Council on Adoptable Children
651-644-3036
www.nacac.org

To learn more go to our web site at:

www.bmtinfonet.org /after/ havingchildren

Chapter Fifteen
PLANNING FOR SURVIVORSHIP

The bone marrow transplant affected my life in every way. I am thankful to wake up each morning. I have learned compassion and empathy for those unable to be 'normal'. I have learned how much it means when others are kind. I have learned the value of a family in my life. I have had a paper on my refrigerator for the last 5 years that reads, 'My goal is to live forever, so far, so good.' The seasons change on our Iowa farm, the crops and animals grow. I, too, hope to keep changing and growing.

Kathleen Jones, ten-year survivor of two transplants

As a survivor of an autologous transplant, you have been through an extraordinary experience. As you move forward with your life, you may find yourself feeling different — different from the people around you and different than your former self.

Survivorship may mean a new appreciation of life, new interests, or new priorities. It also may mean getting used to side effects and learning to function despite them. Although most of these side effects will resolve by the end of the first year after transplant, some survivors must adjust to side effects long-term.

Transplant survivors find joy in the fact that they have been given a new lease on life. However, protecting your health long-term requires a good understanding of the treatment you've undergone and your risk for developing complications later on. It also requires access to healthcare providers who are knowledgeable about transplantation and its late effects, and can monitor you for long-term complications.

Although some patients can return to their transplant center for long-term follow-up care, many cannot. Most primary care physicians and local oncologists have received little or no training in the care of transplant survivors. Thus, you will need a good long-term follow-up plan prepared by your transplant team that outlines your medical history, treatments you received and potential long-term issues that may arise so that your local doctors can provide you with the best care possible.

The symptoms of some complications can resemble other disorders local doctors often see. Without knowledge of your medical background, your local doctor may direct you to specialists or prescribe tests that will miss the actual problem. YOU are an important partner in protecting your health long-term. The more informed you are about your treatment history and risk for long-term complications, the better equipped you will be to advocate for appropriate long-term care.

What Should Be In the Plan?

When you no longer require care at the transplant center, ask your transplant team to prepare a long-term plan for follow-up care. Ideally, your long-term follow-up plan should include the following information:

- the date, dosage and type of chemotherapy you received, including any you received prior to being referred to the transplant center

- the date, type and site of any radiation you received including any you received prior to being referred to the transplant center

- other medications you received while being treated for your disease that have potential long-term health effects

- any serious infections you developed and how they were treated

- if you relapsed after transplant, how it was treated

- potential late effects for each therapy you received including mental health effects

- a list of your medications and allergies

- a list of your vaccinations

- copies of office notes and test results that you can share with your local doctors

- tests and clinical evaluations that should be done periodically to detect possible problems

- who your doctor should contact for questions and instructions

Make several copies of your long-term follow-up plan and be sure to give it to *all* of your doctors, including dentists. Because you have a complicated medical history, you will need to take responsibility for making sure that all of your doc-

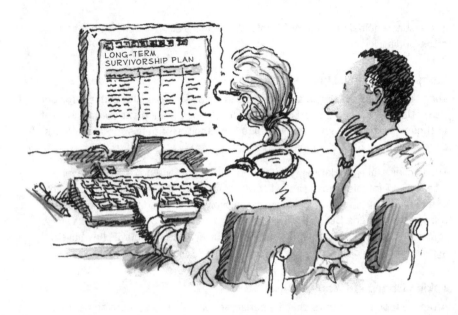

tors know about any medical issues that arise after transplant so that their records are up-to-date. If possible, identify one doctor or nurse practitioner willing and available to coordinate your care so that all the members of your healthcare team are up-to-date on your health history.

Be sure that your transplant team knows the names and contact information for all doctors who are currently caring for you. Update that information annually, particularly if you move or are changing doctors.

Long-Term Follow-Up Care and Tests

Guidelines for long-term follow-up care have been developed by the Center for International Blood and Marrow Transplant Research (CIBMTR), a leading scientific organization that conducts research on blood stem cell transplantation. The guidelines are written in lay language for patients, and include a summary sheet of tests and periodic exams that you should receive which you can give to each of your doctors.

A link to the guidelines can be found on BMT InfoNet's web site at www.bmtinfonet.org/after/protecthealthlongterm.

The Children's Oncology Group has similar guidelines for children who have undergone cancer therapy. These guidelines take into account the effect various chemotherapy drugs and radiation may have on growing children and thus include a number of tests and exams not needed by adults. You can find a link to these guidelines on BMT InfoNet's web site at www.bmtinfonet.org/after/pediatricissues.

Long-Term Follow-Up Clinics

Long-term follow up clinics are available in some areas of the country for cancer patients, and are a good option for autologous transplant survivors. Staff at these centers are specifically trained to monitor patients for late effects of cancer treatment, including a transplant.

These clinics are a relatively new phenomenon and are not available everywhere. BMT InfoNet maintains a list of some survivorship clinics on its web site at www.bmtinfonet.org/after/survivorclinics. If you don't have access to the internet, phone 888-597-7674 for assistance. You can also check with your transplant center or at hospitals in your area to find out if they have a survivorship clinic that can follow you after transplant.

Taking Charge of Your Health

After transplant, patients crave a sense of normalcy. They want to be done with tests, doctors and medical procedures and may become frustrated when setbacks occur.

Setbacks are a normal part of the recovery process. It is not unusual for a patient to be readmitted to the hospital to treat complications that arise after transplant. Be prepared for some ups and downs on the road to recovery. It is best to be cautious. That five minute call to your transplant doctor, or three-day stay in the hospital, while annoying, may save your life.

Be sure to report any mouth sores, weight loss, diarrhea or swelling to your doctor immediately, as these may be signs of problems that need treatment. Protect yourself against sun exposure, check your vitamin D level to protect bone health, and get routine tests such as Pap smears, mammograms and colonoscopies.

Survivors who were transplanted when they were children face additional challenges. Some may not know what treatment they received since they were not the person coordinating care at the time. Check with your parents and your transplant center to get the necessary information to give to your adult healthcare providers. You may require follow-up testing that is not routinely done at adult wellness check-ups, or is normally done at a different stage of life.

You can view an excellent webcast on BMT InfoNet's web site about transitioning from pediatric to adult care after a transplant at www.bmtinfonet.org/webcast under the heading Long-Term Side Effects.

Emotional Well-Being

Emotional distress is common among transplant survivors, at least for awhile. It is a significant problem for caregivers as well.

Stress can be caused by a number of factors. Fear of relapse, changes in body image, the slow rate of recovery, medical setbacks, being socially isolated, financial burdens and not feeling that people really understand what the survivor and their family is going through can create stress even for the most optimistic survivor.

Some survivors find that support groups, on-line chat rooms or ongoing relationships with other survivors provide the best emotional support.

> "They had a reunion at my transplant center last year and a big patient meeting was held. The first thing you know, someone raised her hand and said, 'Has anyone ever experienced such and such problem?' Well, we were off and running. Somebody else said, 'Do you have memory problems?' I described it differently and other people said, 'Yeah, yeah, that's it.' The meeting was a huge success and we all came out grinning because for the first time we were able to get these issues out on the table and get some information about them."

Although face-to-face support groups for transplant survivors are rare, there are online support groups and telephone support programs that many survivors find helpful. BMT InfoNet offers a Caring Connections Program to link patients and family members who need emotional support with others who understand what they are going through. You can request a connection at www.bmtinfonet.org/services/support or by phoning 888-597-7674.

The Association of Cancer Online Resources (ACOR) maintains a discussion list for transplant patients and survivors that many people find helpful. You can access it at www.acor.org. Select the list BMT-Talk.

BMT Support (www.bmtsupport.org) holds weekly chat rooms online for patients and family caregivers. The discussion is moderated by a nurse and BMT survivor.

The services of a psychiatrist, psychologist, social worker or other counselor help some survivors get back a sense of well-being.

> "Fifteen months later when I ended the counseling sessions, I thanked the psychiatrist and told him, 'My transplant doctor gave me back my life, but you put the quality back in my life.'"

Some survivors experience "survivor guilt". It may happen when another transplant patient they know relapses or does not survive the transplant. Support groups, counseling and clergy can be good sources for sorting out these feelings.

Fear of relapse is a major concern, particularly during the early years after transplant. It may take a long time before you are able to make long-term plans or spend a day without thinking about your disease or treatment.

Spouses and Children

Marriages often change after transplant. Some couples report that their relationship is the same or better than before the transplant. For others the opposite is true.

> "Without a doubt, going through the transplant strengthened our marital relationship. We threw out all the trash that had accumulated over the years and got our priorities straight."

> "After my transplant, I changed in ways that my wife couldn't understand. I wanted to go a million miles an hour and experience everything. Activities and friends that were now very important to me seemed trivial to her. Our marriage finally ended in divorce last fall."

> "The whole experience frightened my husband no end. You don't realize how hard it is on the spouse until it's all over. He doesn't want to talk about it, think about it or hear about it. I couldn't even get him to congratulate me on my transplant anniversary. Don't get me wrong, he's a great guy and we love each other very much. But it would be nice to be able to talk with him about the experience sometimes."

Relationships with children can also change after transplant.

> "The transplant was very hard on my daughters who were sixteen, thirteen and two at the time. They were terrified of losing their mother, and each of them showed their stress in a different way. The oldest felt responsible for the younger two if I died, and that was a big burden for someone her age. Even after I came home, my middle one was afraid that I would be sick again, and didn't know how to talk about her fears. The little one literally clung to me for two years. Working through these problems was a long ordeal, but they've all grown to be very mature, responsible kids. I'm very proud of them and they're proud of me."

It may be useful to seek the help of a family therapist to work through strained relationships and enable each party to understand the other person's perspective. Keeping the lines of communication open is key.

Fatigue

Chronic fatigue is a common complaint following transplant. It can interfere with mood, physical activity, and sleep. Unlike the fatigue we experience in everyday life, rest does not always relieve it.

Fatigue can be caused by a number of factors including:

- anemia

- depression

- pain

- sleep disorders

- electrolyte disturbances

- infection

- poorly functioning immune system

- thyroid disorder or other hormone deficiencies

- adrenal insufficiency

- malnutrition

- dehydration

- lack of exercise

- stress

- medications that act on the brain and spinal cord

Survivors who experience fatigue after transplant have decreased energy, a generalized weakness and/or decreased motivation. They may suffer from insomnia or sleep too much, and may wake up tired.

Fatigue can cause sadness, frustration and irritability. It can make it difficult to perform daily tasks and affect memory.

Be sure to report chronic fatigue to your healthcare team. There are a number of tests that can be performed to check for problems like anemia, thyroid problems or adrenal insufficiency which are easily treated.

Getting sufficient sleep is important, but try to avoid sleeping too much as that can decrease your energy. If you nap during the day, try to limit it to one hour so that you sleep well at night.

Exercise and physical activity can also improve symptoms of fatigue. Even five to ten minutes of exercise several times daily can help.

Drinking sufficient liquids and consuming enough carbohydrates and protein are important tools in managing fatigue. If need be, your transplant team can refer you to a nutritionist who can help develop a plan tailored to your needs.

Think of ways to conserve your energy for the times of the day that you need it most. Sit down when bathing or preparing meals. Plan to do necessary activities at the time of day when you have the most energy. Pace yourself, avoid rushing and delegate responsibilities when possible.

If fatigue interferes with your ability to work, consider talking with your employer about alternate ways to manage your workload. Set realistic goals, perhaps shorten hours or request a disability leave of absence. Don't be embarrassed to ask for help. Organizations such as the Cancer Legal Resource Center or the Patient Advocate Foundation can help you understand your legal rights if you need to take time off work. You can find links to these organizations at www.bmtinfonet/after/finances.

BMT offers several excellent webcasts on managing fatigue. Go to www.bmtinfonet.org/webcast and scroll down to Fatigue.

Cognitive Changes

Many survivors find that their memory is not as sharp as it used to be, or that organizing activities or learning new tasks are more difficult. This is sometimes referred to as "chemobrain", and while the problem is short-term for most survivors, for some it is an ongoing concern that can affect their work and daily living.

Cognitive changes can be caused by a number of factors. These include:

- chemotherapy or radiation you received prior to transplant
- pain medications and psychiatric medications
- anticonvulsants
- insomnia and sleep medications
- fatigue
- anemia
- kidney or liver problems
- psychological distress
- premature menopause

Cognitive problems should be discussed with your transplant team. After ruling out possible causes such as infection, anemia, poor sleep or emotional distress, the team may refer you to a neuropsychologist for an evaluation. The psychologist may suggest strategies to compensate for the problem such as making lists, using post-it notes as reminders, pill boxes with your necessary medications for each day of the week, reducing distractions such as large crowds, and changes in sleep and exercise routine.

Some survivors have found that medications such as Ritalin®, Provigil®, Aricept® or Namenda® have helped with cognitive challenges. More research is needed to enable scientists to understand why survivors often experience "chemobrain" and find ways to prevent and manage it.

BMT InfoNet offers several webcasts on learning and memory problems after transplant pertaining to both children and adult survivors. To learn more go to www.bmtinfonet.org/webcast and scroll down to Learning & Memory Problems.

The Bottom Line

It may take a while before the constant worrying about your health is over for both you and your loved ones. While physical well-being is important, strong family relationships, friendships, inner spirituality and helping others are also important factors that make for a good quality of life. Many survivors feel the transplant experience helped them get their priorities straight and prompted them to live each day to the fullest, rather than put off the important things for the future.

Many say the experience taught them a lot about what their bodies and minds are capable of doing. Prior to the transplant, everyone is frightened of potential physical complications and pain, and most survivors experience emotional ups and downs for many months following the transplant. Yet, they find ways to cope with these problems and enjoy their second chance at life.

> "It took almost two years for me to adjust and reshape my life. It required counseling, support group meetings, constant family support, the loyalty and help from friends and a renewed faith in God. I am now a reasonably happy and content survivor. I've gained peace of mind and peace of soul. I'm finally getting a glimpse of who I really am, and I like what I'm seeing. I still have lingering complications, but if I never feel any better physically than I do right now, I'll still count my blessings. The transplant was indeed a traumatic experience, but it gave me the only chance I had to live, and I'm glad that I took it."

To learn more go to our web site at:

www.bmtinfonet.org/after/top

Appendix A

ABOUT
BLOOD CELLS

Blood is composed of many different kinds of cells, each with a specific function. Most blood cells are formed in the bone marrow and released into the bloodstream at various stages of maturity. In healthy adults, an estimated 500 million new blood cells are produced each hour.

During your treatment, the medical team will be monitoring the level of various types of blood cells. Those that you will hear about most often are red blood cells, white blood cells and platelets.

Red blood cells (erythrocytes) pick up oxygen in the lungs and transport it to tissues throughout the body. They also pick up carbon dioxide from tissues, and transport it back to the lungs where it is exhaled.

White blood cells (leukocytes) are needed to fight infection. The main types of white blood cells and their functions are described on the next page.

Platelets (thrombocytes) are the smallest cell elements in the bloodstream. Platelets are needed to control bleeding.

All blood cells evolve from primitive cells in the marrow called pluripotent stem cells. Pluripotent stem cells are unique cells that can replicate themselves as well as produce two other types of stem cells called myeloid stem cells and lymphoid stem cells. These stem cells, in turn, either replicate themselves or produce other cells that eventually evolve into blood cells. A group of white blood cells called lymphocytes evolve from lymphoid stem cells. Red blood cells, platelets and other types of white blood cells evolve from the myeloid stem cell.

White Blood Cells

There are five main types of white blood cells: lymphocytes, monocytes, neutrophils, eosinophils and basophils.

Lymphocytes are the smallest white blood cells. Lymphocytes fight viral infections and help destroy bacteria, fungi and other parasites. One type — the T-cell —is the body's main defense against viruses and protozoa. A second type — the B-cell — produces proteins called antibodies. The antibodies attach to the surface of foreign organisms or the cells they've invaded. They then summon another group of proteins, called "complement" to surround the organism or infected cell and dissolve a hole in it.

Monocytes are the largest white blood cells. They can surround and destroy invading bacteria and fungi. They also clean up the debris that is left after other white blood cells destroy foreign organisms. When monocytes leave the bloodstream and enter tissues or organs, they can evolve into larger cells called macrophages. Macrophages have an even greater ability to destroy foreign organisms that invade the body.

Neutrophils (also called granulocytes) fight bacterial infections. They patrol the body via the blood stream or lymph system, seeking out and destroying harmful bacteria. (The lymph system is a network of vessels that run alongside the blood stream.)

Eosinophils attack protozoa that cause infection.

Basophils are the least common type of white blood cell and their function is not completely understood. They play an important role in regulating allergic reactions such as asthma, hives, hay fever and reactions to drugs.

Blast Cells

White blood cells pass through several stages of development before maturing into lymphocytes, monocytes, neutrophils, eosinophils or basophils. Very immature white blood cells are called blast cells or blasts.

Blast cells are usually found only in the bone marrow. If a large number of blast cells are detected in the bloodstream, the patient most likely has leukemia. A smaller number of blasts are sometimes detected in the bloodstream of patients who are recovering from chemotherapy or an infection. This is common and is *not* an indication that the patient has leukemia.

UNDERSTANDING BLOOD TESTS

Have you ever wondered what all those blood tests were measuring? Here's a guide to help you make sense of the results.

Complete Blood Count (CBC)

Describes the number, type and form of each blood cell. It includes all tests described below.

Red Blood Cell Count (RBC)

Counts the number of red blood cells in a single drop (a microliter) of blood. Normal ranges vary according to age and sex.

Men:	4.5 to 6.2 million
Women:	4.2 to 5.4 million
Children:	4.6 to 4.8 million

A low RBC count may indicate anemia, excess body fluid, or hemorrhaging. A high RBC count may indicate polycythemia (an excessive number of red blood cells in the blood) or dehydration.

Total Hemoglobin Concentration

Hemoglobin gives red blood cells their color and carries oxygen from the lungs to cells. This test measures the grams of hemoglobin in a deciliter (100 ml) of blood, which can help physicians determine the severity of anemia or polycythemia.

Normal values are:

Men:	14 to 18 g/dl
Women:	12 to 16 g/dl
Children:	11 to 13 g/dl

A significant anemia occurs when the hemoglobin drops below 10 g/dl.

Hematocrit

Hematocrit measures the percentage of red blood cells in the sample. Normal values vary greatly:

Men:	45% to 57%
Women:	37% to 47%
Children:	36% to 40%

Erythrocyte (RBC) Indices

Three indices that measure the number, size of red blood cells and amount of hemoglobin contained in each. Mean corpuscular volume (MCV) measures the volume of red blood cells. Normal is 84 to 99 fl. Mean corpuscular hemoglobin (MCH) measures the amount of hemoglobin in an average cell. Normal is 26 to 32 pg. Mean corpuscular hemoglobin concentration (MCHC) measures the concentration of hemoglobin in red blood cells. Normal is 30% to 36%.

White Blood Cell Count (WBC)

Measures the number of white blood cells in a drop (microliter) of blood. Normal values range from 4,100 to 10,900 but can be altered greatly by factors such as exercise, stress and disease. A low WBC may indicate viral infection or toxic reaction. A high WBC count may indicate infection, leukemia, or tissue damage. An increased risk of infection occurs once the WBC drops below 1,000/microliter, and especially below 500/microliter.

WBC Differential

Determines the percentage of each type of white blood cell in the sample. Multiplying the percentage by the total count of white blood cells indicates the actual number of each type of white blood cell in the sample. Normal values are:

Type	Percentage	Number
Neutrophil	50-60%	3,000-7,000
Eosinophils	1-4%	50-400
Basophils	0.5 - 2%	25-100
Lymphocytes	20-40%	1,000-4,000
Monocytes	2-9%	100-600

A serious infection can develop once the total neutrophil count (percentage of neutrophils times total WBC) drops below 500/microliter.

Platelet Count

Measures the number of platelets in a drop (microliter) of blood. Platelet counts increase during strenuous activity and in certain conditions called myeloproliferative disorders. Infections, inflammations, malignancies and removal of the spleen can also cause platelet counts to increase. Platelet counts decrease just before menstruation. Normal values range from 150,000 to 400,000 per microliter. A count below 50,000 can result in spontaneous bleeding; below 10,000, patients are at risk of severe, life-threatening bleeding.

GLOSSARY OF TERMS

This glossary contains terms and abbreviations you may encounter during your treatment that are not explained elsewhere in this book.

ABW: Actual body weight.

Acute: Having severe symptoms and a short course.

Adjuvant therapy: Additional drug or other treatment designed to enhance the effectiveness of the primary treatment.

ADR: Adverse drug reaction.

ALC: Absolute lymphocyte count.

Alkaline phosphatase: An enzyme produced by the liver or bone.

ALL: Acute lymphoblastic leukemia.

Allergen: Any substance that causes an allergy.

Allergy: An inappropriate and harmful response of the immune system to normally harmless substances.

Alopecia: Loss of hair.

AML: Acute myeloid leukemia or acute myelogenous leukemia.

Anaphylaxis: Acute allergic reaction that causes shortness of breath, rash, wheezing, hypotension.

Anaphylactic shock: A life-threatening allergic reaction characterized by a swelling of body tissues including the throat, difficulty in breathing, and a sudden fall in blood pressure.

ANC: Absolute neutrophil count.

Anemia: Too few red blood cells in the bloodstream, resulting in insufficient oxygen to tissues and organs.

Anorexia: Loss of appetite.

Antibiotic: A drug used to fight bacterial infections.

Antibody: A protein produced by the body, in response to the presence of a foreign substance, that fights the invading organism.

Antiemetic: A drug used to control nausea and vomiting.

Antigen: A substance that evokes a response from the body's immune system resulting in the production of antibodies or other defensive action by white blood cells.

Antiserum: Serum that contains antibodies.

Antitoxins: Antibodies that inactivate toxins produced by certain bacteria.

Apheresis: A procedure by which blood is withdrawn from a patient's arm and circulated through a machine that removes certain components and returns the remaining components to the patient. This procedure is used to remove platelets from platelet donors' blood, or stem cells from patients undergoing a stem cell harvest.

APL: Acute promyelocytic leukemia.

Aplasia: A failure to develop or form. In bone marrow aplasia, the marrow cavity is empty.

Ascites: Accumulation of fluid in the stomach area.

Ataxia: Loss of balance.

Autoantibody: An antibody that reacts against a person's own tissue.

Autograft: Bone marrow or stem cells removed from the patient to be used in an autologous transplant.

Autoimmune disease: A disease that results when the immune system attacks the body's own tissues.

Baseline test: Test that measures an organ's normal level of functioning. Used to determine if any changes in organ function occur following treatment.

Biological response modifiers: Substances, either natural or man made, that boost, direct, or restore normal immune defenses.

Biopsy: Removal of tissue for examination under a microscope, sometimes required to enable the doctor to make a proper diagnosis.

Blast crisis: In patients with chronic myelogenous leukemia, the progression of the disease to an advanced phase, evidenced by an increased number of immature white blood cells in the circulating blood. Sometimes loosely used to describe a rapid increase in the white blood cell count of any leukemic patient.

BM: Bone marrow.

BMSC: Bone marrow stem cell.

BMT: Bone marrow transplant. Also used as an abbreviation for blood and marrow transplant

BRM: Biological response modifier.

Calorie: A measure of energy your body gets from food.

Carbohydrate: One of the three nutrients that supply calories (energy) to the body.

Cardiac: Pertaining to the heart.

Catheter: Small, flexible plastic tube inserted into a portion of the body to administer or remove fluids.

CBSC: Cord blood stem cell.

Central line: Central venous catheter.

Central venous catheter: Small, flexible plastic tube inserted into the large vein above the heart, through which drugs and blood products can be given, and blood samples withdrawn.

Chemo: Chemotherapy.

Chemo-responsive: Responds to chemotherapy. For example, a tumor is chemo-responsive if it shrinks in size following chemotherapy.

Chemotherapy: Drug or combination of drugs designed to kill cancerous cells.

Chromosomes: Physical structures in the cell's nucleus that house the genes. Each human cell has 23 pairs of chromosomes.

Chronic: Persisting for a long time.

CLL: Chronic lymphocytic leukemia.

CML: Chronic myeloid leukemia or chronic myelogenous leukemia.

CMMOL: Chronic myelomonocytic leukemia.

CNS: Central nervous system.

Conjunctivitis: Eye inflammation.

Contracture: Shortening of muscle, skin and other soft tissue, usually in the limbs.

CP: Chronic phase.

CPR: Cardio pulmonary resuscitation.

CR: Complete remission.

Cryopreservation: To preserve by freezing at very low temperatures.

CSF: Colony stimulating factor.

CT scan: Also called a CAT scan or CT-X-ray. A three-dimensional x-ray.

Cytogenetic remission: (see Remission, cytogenetic.)

Cytokines: Powerful chemical substances secreted by cells. They play an important role in regulating the immune system.

DC: Dendritic cell.

Dendritic: Rare but important cells that spur T-Cells into action.

Dermatitis: A skin rash.

DFS: Disease free survival.

DNA (deoxyribonucleic acid): Nucleic acid that is found in the cell nucleus and that is the carrier of genetic information.

Dysgeusia: Changes in the way foods are perceived to taste.

Dysphasia: Difficulty swallowing.

Dysplasia: Alteration in the size, shape and organization of cells or tissues.

ECG: Electrocardiogram.

-ectomy: Surgical removal. For example, spleenectomy is surgical removal of the spleen.

Edema: Abnormal accumulation of fluid. For example, pulmonary edema refers to a build-up of fluid in the lungs.

EFS: Event-free survival.

EKG: Electrocardiogram.

Electrocardiogram: Test to determine the pattern of a patient's heartbeat.

Electrolyte: Minerals found in the blood such as potassium that must be maintained within a certain range to prevent organ malfunction.

Emesis: Vomiting.

-emia: Of the blood. Usually refers to a blood disorder, e.g., leukemia or anemia.

Encephalopathy: Abnormal functioning of the brain.

Enzyme: A protein that is capable of triggering a chemical reaction.

Esophagitis: Inflammation of the throat.

Febrile: Pertaining to fever.

Foley catheter: Flexible plastic tube inserted into the bladder to provide continuous urinary drainage.

Gastritis: Inflammation of the stomach.

Gastrointestinal: Refers to the stomach and intestines.

Gene: A unit of genetic material that carries the directions a cell uses to perform a specific function, such as making a given protein.

Glucose: A sugar found in blood.

Hb: Hemoglobin.

HBV: Hepatitis B virus.

HCT: Hematopoietic cell transplantation.

HCV: Hepatitis C virus.

HD: Hodgkin Disease.

Hematology: The study of blood and its disorders.

Hematopoiesis: The formation and development of blood cells, usually takes place in the bone marrow.

Hematopoietic cells: Cells from which all blood cells derive.

Hemoglobin: The part of red blood cells that carries oxygen to tissues.

Hemorrhage: Bleeding.

Hemorrhagic cystitis: Bladder ulcers.

Hepat (o): Pertaining to the liver.

HHV6: Human herpes virus 6.

HLA: Human leukocyte antigen.

Hyper-: Excessive, increased.

Hyperal: Hyperalimentation.

Hyperpigmentation: Darkening of the skin.

Hypertension: High blood pressure.

Hypo-: A deficiency, less than usual.

Hypotension: Low blood pressure.

i.m.: intramuscular.

Immune complex: A cluster of interlocking antigens and antibodies.

Immune response: The reactions of the immune system to foreign substances.

Immunocompetent: Capable of developing an immune response.

Immunocompromised: A condition in which the immune system is not functioning normally.

Immunoglobulin: An antibody.

Immunosuppression: A condition in which the patient's immune system is functioning at a lower than normal level.

Immunotoxin: A naturally occurring toxin.

Inflammatory response: Redness, warmth, swelling, pain, and loss of function produced in response to infection, as the result of increased blood flow and an influx of immune cells and secretions.

Interleukins: A major group of lymphokines and monokines.

Intramuscular: Within a muscle.

Intravenous: In a vein.

IP: Interstitial pneumonia.

- itis: Inflammation.

IV: Intravenous.

Karnofsky performance score: A measure of the patient's overall physical health, judged by his level of activity.

KPS: Karnofsky performance score.

Lactose intolerance: An inability to easily digest lactose.

Lactose: A sugar found in milk.

LAK cells: Lymphocytes transformed in the laboratory into lymphokine-activated killer cells, which attack tumor cells.

Laminar air flow unit: An air-filtering system used at some transplant facilities to remove particulate matter and fungi from the air.

Lipids: Fats.

Low-microbial diet: Special diet designed to reduce a patient's exposure to bacteria.

Lymph nodes: Small bean-shaped organs of the immune system, distributed widely throughout the body.

Lymph: A transparent, slightly yellow fluid that carries lymphocytes, bathes the body tissues, and drains into the lymphatic vessels.

Lymphatic vessels: A body-wide network of channels, similar to the blood vessels, which transport lymph to the immune organs and into the bloodstream.

Lymphoid organs: The organs of the immune system, where lymphocytes develop and congregate. They include the bone marrow, thymus, lymph nodes, spleen, and various other clusters of lymphoid tissue. The blood vessels and lymphatic vessels can also be considered lymphoid organs.

Lymphokines: Powerful chemical substances secreted by lymphocytes. These soluble molecules help direct and regulate the immune responses.

Mab: Monoclonal antibody.

Malabsorption: Failure of intestines to properly absorb oral medications or nutrients from food.

MDS: Myelodysplastic syndrome.

Mentation: Thinking.

Metabolite: A by-product of the breakdown of either food or medication by the body.

Metastatic: Spread of a disease from the organ or tissue of origin to another part of the body.

Microbes: Minute living organisms, including bacteria, viruses, fungi and protozoa.

Microorganisms: Microscopic plants or animals.

Minerals: Nutrients required by the body in small amounts to maintain proper fluid balance and body function.

MM: Multiple myeloma.

Molecule: The smallest amount of a specific chemical substance that can exist alone.

Monoclonal antibodies: Antibodies that are all identical, derived from a single source.

Monokines: Powerful chemical substances secreted by some white blood cells. These soluble molecules help direct and regulate the immune responses.

Morbidity: Sickness, side effects and symptoms of a treatment or disease.

MRD: Minimal residual disease.

MRI: Magnetic resonance imaging. A method of taking pictures of body tissue using magnetic fields and radio waves.

MTD: Maximum tolerated dose.

Myeloablative: Suppresses the immune system

Natural Killer cells: Type of white blood cell that can recognize and destroy some tumor cells

Nephro-: Pertaining to the kidneys.

Neuro-: Pertaining to the nervous system.

NHL: Non-Hodgkin lymphoma.

NPO: Do not take anything by mouth.

Nutrient: The part of food you eat that's used by the body to grow, function and stay alive.Nutrients include protein, carbohydrate, minerals, fat and vitamins.

Oncology: The study of cancer.

Opportunistic infection: An infection in a person whose immune system is suppressed, caused by an organism that does not usually trouble people with healthy immune systems.

Organism: An individual living thing.

Oto-: Pertaining to the ear.

Packed red blood cells: Whole blood minus the plasma.

Palliative: Provides relief rather than a cure.

Pancytopenia: A deficiency of all types of blood cells.

Parasite: A plant or animal that lives, grows and feeds on or within another living organism.

Passive immunity: Immunity resulting from the transfer of antibodies or antiserum produced by another individual.

-pathy: Disease.

PBPC: Peripheral blood progenitor cells.

PBSC: Peripheral blood stem cells.

-penia: Deficiency. For example, neutropenia means a deficiency of a type of white blood cell called a neutrophil.

Petechiae: Small red spots on the skin that usually indicate a low platelet count.

Ph: Philadelphia chromosome.

Phlebitis: Inflammation of a vein.

-plasia: Development, formation.

PLT: Platelet.

PR: Partial remission.

Prognosis: The predicted or likely outcome.

Prophylactic: Preventive measure or medication.

Protein: One of the three nutrients that supply calories to the body. Protein helps build muscle, bone, skin and blood.

Protocol: The plan for treating the patient.

Pulmonary: Pertaining to the lungs.

QOL: Quality of life.

Reflux: A backflow of acid from the stomach into the esophagus.

Relapse: Recurrence of the disease following treatment.

Relapse-free survival: Survival after treatment without relapse.

Remission, complete: Condition in which no cancerous cells can be detected by a microscope, and the patient appears to be disease-free.

Remission, cytogenetic: In persons who had a chromosomal abnormality, a remission with normal chromosomes.

Remission, partial: Generally means that by all methods used to measure the existence of a tumor, there has been at least a 50 percent regression of the disease following treatment.

Renal: Pertaining to the kidney.

RFS: Relapse-free survival.

RNA (ribonucleic acid): A nucleic acid that is found in the cytoplasm and also in the nucleus of some cells. One function of RNA is to direct the production of proteins.

RSV: Respiratory syncytial virus.

s.c.: Subcutaneous.

SCLC: Small cell lung cancer.

Sepsis: The presence of organisms in the blood.

Serum: The clear liquid that separates from the blood when it is allowed to clot. This fluid retains any antibodies that were present in the whole blood.

Solid tumor: A cancer that originates in organ or tissue other than bone marrow or the lymph system.

Spleen: A lymphoid organ in the abdominal cavity that is an important center for immune system activities.

Stomatitis: Inflammation of the mouth, tongue or gums.

Subcutaneous: Under the skin.

Superinfection: An infection that occurs in a patient who already has a different type of infection.

Tandum transplant: Two planned transplants, one after another.

TBI: Total body irradiation.

Thymus: A primary lymphoid organ, high in the chest, where lymphocytes proliferate and mature.

TLC: Total lung capacity.

Toxins: Agents produced by plants and bacteria normally very damaging to human cells.

Trauma: Injury.

Tumor burden: The size of the tumor or number of abnormal cells in the organ or tissue.

Tumor: Uncontrolled growth of abnormal cells in an organ or tissue.

Ultrasound: A technique for taking a picture of internal organs or other structures using sound waves.

URI: Upper respiratory infection.

Vaccine: A substance that contains components of an infectious organism. Injecting the vaccine into a person will stimulate an immune response (but not a full case of disease), and protect the person against subsequent infection by that organism.

Whole blood: Blood that has not been separated into its various components.

Xerostomia: Dryness of the mouth caused by malfunctioning salivary glands.

INDEX

Acyclovir, 61-62

Adenovirus, 63, 70

Adoption, 111, 113-114

Alkaline phosphatase, 69, 131

Alopecia (see also Hair loss), 131

American Association of Sexual Educators Counselors and Therapists, 10

American Society for Reproductive Medicine, 113

American Society for Blood and Marrow Transplantation (see ASBMT), 19

Amphotericin B, 61, 69

Anemia, 127, 131, 134

Antibody, 132, 136-137

Antidepressant, 33

Antiemetic, 55, 132

Appetite
  lack of, 79

Arrhythmia, 57

Artificial insemination, 111-112

ASBMT (see American Society for Blood and Marrow Transplantation), 19

Ascites, 132

Aspergillus, 61

Ativan®, 88

B-cell, 126

Bacterial infection (see infection, bacterial), 60

Bactrim®, 78, 63

Basophils, 126, 128

Be the Match®, 3

Bile, 67-68, 70-71

Bile duct, 67-68, 71

Biliary disease, 71

Bilirubin, 56, 67-68, 70

Bladder irritation, 56

Blast cell, 126, 132

Blood counts, 9-10, 127

Blood tests, 127-129

Bone marrow, 5, 6

Bone marrow harvest, 8-9

Breathing problems, 56

Busulfan, 53, 55, 57

Candida, 60-61, 69

Caregivers, 46, 95-105

Carmustine, 55, 57

Cataracts, 57

Catheter, 56, 133

   Central venous, 133

   Foley catheter, 135

CBC, 127

Central venous, 133

Chemotherapy,

   high-dose, 1-3, 6

   side effects, 6-7, 31-32, 54-58

   bladder, 56

   cataracts, 57

   confusion, 57

   dental problems, 58

   growth delayed, 57, 58

   hair loss, 54-55

   heart problems, 57

   learning disability, 58, 122-123

   liver problems, 56

   lung problems, 56

   mouth dry, 76

   mouth sores, 29, 31, 55, 75-76, 87-88,

   muscle spasms, cramping, 57

Electrolytes, 57

Emotional stress, 11, 16
  caregiving and, 97-98, 119
  children and, 10, 16, 43-44, 123
  managing, 11, 27-28, 32-33, 97-98, 119-120

Engraftment, 9

Eosinophil, 126

Epstein-Barr virus, 63, 70

ERISA, 23

Erythrocyte (see also Red blood cells), 128

Erythrocyte indices, 128

Etoposide, 55

Eucerin®, 88

Event-free survival, 18, 134

Eye, 55, 62, 64, 133
  Infection, 62-64

FACT (see Foundation for Accreditation of Cellular Therapy), 14

Famciclovir, 62

Fatigue, 121-122

Feeding, intravenous, 55, 70-71, 75, 136

Fertilehope.org, 113

Fertility post-transplant, 42, 111-113

Filgrastim, 7

Fluconazole, 61, 69

Fluid retention, 56

Foley catheter, 135

Foundation for Accreditation of Cellular Therapy, 14

Fundraising, 26

Fungal infection (see Infection, fungal), 60-61

Fungi, 59-61, 64, 69, 126

Gallbladder, 67, 71

Gallstones, 68, 71

Ganciclovir, 61, 63

G-CSF (see filgrastim), 7

Granulocyte (neutrophil), 126, 128

Growth, delayed in children, 57-58

Hair loss, 29, 31, 54-55, 109

Life insurance, 24-26

Liver, 56-57

  biliary disease, 71

  blood test abnormalities, 56, 68

  damage, 68-69

  disorders, 67-71

  enzymes, 56, 68, 70

  function of, 67

  infection, 63-64, 68-69

  veno-occlusive disease, 68-69, 84

Long-term survivors (see Survival long-term), 115-123

Lumbar puncture, 88

Lung, 56-57

  damage, 56-57

  infection, 60-61, 63-64, 68-70

  pressure on, 68-69

Lymphocyte (see also White blood cell), 125-126, 128, 136

Malabsorption, 137

Marital stress, 47

Massage, 84, 90, 92

MCH (see also Mean corpuscular hemoglobin), 128

MCHC (see also Mean corpuscular hemoglobin concentration), 128

MCV (see also Mean corpuscular volume), 128

Mean corpuscular hemoglobin (see also MCH), 128

Mean corpuscular hemoglobin concentration (see also MCHC), 128

Mean corpuscular volume (see also MCV), 128

Megace®, 79

Memory problems, 58, 122-123

Menopause, premature, 57, 109

MESNA®, 56

Monoclonal antibodies, 8, 137

Monocyte, 126, 128

Morphine, 84, 87-88

Motrin®, 84

Mouth, 10-11, 31, 54-55, 59-60, 76-77

  dry, 76-77

  side effects, 31-32, 55,

  sores, 31, 55, 62, 75-75, 87-88

Mucositis (see Mouth sores), 55
Muscle, 73, 91, 136
  cramping, 7, 57
  infection, 64
  spasms, 57
  tightness, 55

National Association of Insurance Commissioners (NAIC), 25
National Marrow Donor Registry, 3
Natural killer cell, 138
Nausea, 54-55, 78-79
Nerve damage (see also Numbness Tingling), 57
Neutropenia, 59, 138
Neutrophil, 69, 128-129
Numbness, 57
  feet, 57
  hands, 57
  lips, 7
Nutrition, 74-81
  calories needed by patients, 73
  changing diet, 73
  parenteral (see Feeding intravenous), 75

Opioid, 78, 80, 84, 88-89
Organ damage (see also specific organs), 56

Pain, 83-88
Papovavirus, 63
Patient controlled analgesia machine, 87
PCA (see patient controlled analgesia machine), 87
Pediatric transplant, 39-51
  behavioral problems after, 49
  concerns of siblings, 41, 46-47, 49
  dental problems after, 58
  growth problems after, 58
  learning disabilities after, 58
  preparing child for medical procedures, 45-46
Pentamidine, 63
Platelets, 5, 125

definition, 125

donating, 34

counts, 129

transfusion, 9, 10

Pluripotent stem cell, 125

Pneumocystis carinii, 63

Pneumonia, 56, 61, 63, 136

bacterial, 60

fungal, 60-61

protozoan, 63-64

viral, 63

Preparative regimen (see also Chemotherapy high-dose) (see also Total body irradiation), 9, 53-58

Protocol, 17, 139

Protozoa, 63-64

Quality of life after transplant, 12, 123

Radiation (see Total body irradiation), 73

RBC, 127-128

Recovery period,

long-term, 115-123

short-term, 11-12

Red blood cell, 125

Red blood cell count, 127-128

Relapse,

fear of, 119-120

Reproduction after transplant, 111-113

Reproductive organs,

damage to, 57

Respiratory syncitial virus, 63

Ribavirin, 63, 70

RSV (see Respiratory syncitial virus), 63, 139

Saliva, 76-78

stimulate production of, 76

thick, 77-78

Sedation, conscious, 88

Sedatives, 33, 54, 70

Septra® (see also Trimethoprim/sulfamethoxazole), 63, 78

Severe combined immunodeficiency syndrome, 3

Sexuality after transplant, 107-110

Shingles (see Varicella zoster virus), 62-63

Skin, 55-56

    dark spots, 56

    infection, 59-60, 62

    irradiated, 92

    patch, 87

    rash (see also dermatitis), 55, 134

    yellowing (see Jaundice), 56

Sleeplessness (see also insomnia), 33

Sperm banking, 111-112

Stem cell, 1-3

    apheresis (see also Stem cell harvest), 7, 132

    engraftment, 9

    harvest, 7

    types of, 125

Stress, 11, 16

    caregiver, 91, 96

    emotional, 119-120

    marital, 47-48

    side effects, 31, 32

Success rates, 17-18

Support groups, 36, 119

Survival long-term, 115-123

Survivor guilt, 119

Swallowing painful (see Throat sores), 11, 87-88

Syngeneic transplant, 2

Taste change in (also see Eating Problems), 77

TBI (see Total body irradiation), 73

T-cell, 126

Teeth, 55, 58

Thiotepa, 55

Throat sores, 55, 62, 75-76

Thrombocytes (see Platelets), 125

Tingling in hands and feet, 57

Total body irradiation, 73

White blood cells (see also B-cell, T-cell, lymphocyte, monocyte, neutrophil, eosinophil, basophil), 125, 126

White blood cell count, 128

Work after transplant, 11

Did You Find This Book Helpful?

Autologous Stem Cell Transplants: A Handbook for Patients is published by BMT InfoNet – a not-for-profit organization dedicated to helping families cope with the transplant experience.

BMT InfoNet is funded by contributions from people, like you, who understand how important it is to have reliable information and support before, during and after transplant.

It's not possible to pay back all of the wonderful people who have supported you through your transplant, but you can pay it forward!

Your tax-deductible gift to BMT InfoNet will help others facing a bone marrow, stem cell or cord blood transplant navigate the transplant journey.

You can donate online at www.bmtinfonet.org/donate or make a pledge by phoning 888-597-7674. Whether you have $5 or $50,000 to give, your gift will make a huge difference in someone's life.

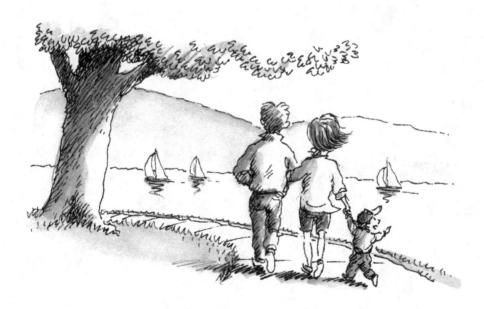

Notes

Autologous Stem Cell Transplants: A Handbook for Patients